MW01612707

HEAL+H
CHEQUE

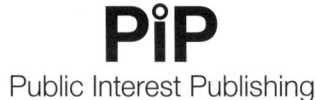

PiP
Public Interest Publishing

HEAL✝H
CHEQUE

The truth we should all know about
New Zealand's public health system

Gareth Morgan
& Geoff Simmons
with John McCrystal

ACKNOWLEDGEMEN⁺S

The book has benefited greatly from the input of a wide range of people, particularly from professionals working within New Zealand's healthcare sector. To all those interviewed – and we're conscious the interviews were full and at times fatiguing for the interviewees – we extend our sincere thanks. Without that feedback from those at the coalface, we would not have got an adequate picture – the literature can only provide so much. In particular, thanks go to Jackie Cumming at Victoria University, Stephen Streat from Auckland Hospital and Robin Gauld at Otago University for their expert and timely advice.

Once compiled, the task of communicating the messages from this study to a reading public is anything but trivial and once again we'd like to thank John McCrystal for crafting the vast array of detail into a form that weaves a story while not losing the essence. His patience and on this occasion accommodation of the totally unreasonable deadlines we requested has been exemplary.

To the team at Phantom Books who have taken the manuscript and created the book as you have it – also to unreasonable deadlines – our thanks are also extended. This project has been funded by the Morgan Family Charitable Foundation (http://www.morgancharity.org/) as part of its public education programme, and the authors thank the Foundation for making the study possible.

Finally all errors and omissions are of course our own.

Designed by Typeface.
Printed in Auckland, New Zealand by McCollams.
First published in 2009 by The Public Interest Publishing Company Ltd (PiP).

Enquiries to Phantom House Publishing:
Fax: +64 4 384 5451
Email: info@phantomhouse.com
Web: www.phantomhouse.com

Copyright © 2009 by Morgan Family Charitable Trust.
All rights reserved; no part of the contents of this book may be reproduced in any form without the permission of the publisher.

ISBN 978-0-9864574-1-8

CONTEN+S

INTRODUC✝ION

'Look to your health,' the author of an influential English textbook on fishing wrote in the middle of the seventeenth century, 'and if you have it, praise god… for health is the second blessing that we mortals are capable of; a blessing that money cannot buy.'

The first blessing, presumably, was the gullibility of fish.

In all that time, nothing much has changed, apart from the fact that health is a now a blessing that money *can* buy, to a limited degree. Four centuries after the good author of *The Compleat Angler* was straying off topic, medicine has advanced to the extent where we can not only hope, but expect to recover from many of the illnesses and afflictions that carried away hapless fishermen back then. Some of the diseases that were the scourge of the early modern world have been all but eradicated – the bubonic plague, for example, and smallpox. Giving birth and being born are nowhere near as hazardous as they once were, and once you're old enough to be given your first fishing rod, you can reasonably expect to be spinning a line for nearly twice as long as your average seventeenth century counterpart. It's all thanks to modern medicine, to the techniques and technologies that our burgeoning scientific understanding has made possible.

'Now don't it always seem to go,' as twentieth century sage Joni Mitchell wrote, 'you don't know what you got till it's gone.' OK, she was writing about a skating rink, but she may just as well have been writing about our health. Because medicine has pushed most of humankind's traditional pathogenic enemies out beyond the circle of the firelight – and can deal with most things that manage to sneak past the cordon – we take our health very much for granted. When we're young, we're bulletproof. As we age, we're confident that drugs and surgery will fix us up if we fall ill. It's only when we're older, and things begin falling irremediably apart that we realise our health is ours for a limited time only, and it's only then that we become aware of its true value. By then, of course, it's too late.

And because of the way we've organised things in this country over the last fifty years (notwithstanding constant reforms and reorganisations in the last thirty), New Zealanders have come to take the public health system for granted, too. Some of us carry private health insurance, and prefer to pay for treatment in a private clinic rather than join a queue in the public system. But those people are the exceptions. For the majority of Kiwis, low-cost healthcare, along with education, an effective police force and justice system, is one of the things we pay taxes for. And as you can tell by the reaction every time it's tampered with, access to healthcare has become even more entrenched in our expectations than the other things we regard as public goods. It's closer these days to an inalienable right rather than part of a renegotiable social contract.

But it's all very well to carry placards and write letters to the editor or your MP or the Minister of Health asserting your right to healthcare. Who is obliged to supply it? Just because the government has traditionally done it doesn't mean it's going to continue to be willing, let alone able to. For as we'll show in this book, the easy presumption that the government will continue to fix us up whenever we're feeling poorly is itself looking increasingly sick.

Like the rest of the developed world, our social systems are currently bracing themselves for the impact of a tsunami of wrinklies, the Geezer Glut that will set in as all those people begotten in the baby boom after the Second World War age.

Thirty years hence, fully a quarter of our population will be aged 65 or above. Since most of us become needier, medically speaking, in our old age – in most Western countries a quarter of the money spent on healthcare is spent in the last two years of life – that's a huge burden imminently about to settle on the shoulders of the existing health system.

And it's not just the boomers who are the problem. As a rule, after the wild years of free love and substance abuse, a large proportion settled down to sober lives of coining it and looking after themselves with macrobiotic diets and aerobic exercise regimes (you only need to look at what gets advertised on telly to see the baby boomer generation's preoccupation with health and well-being shining through). Pity about their kids and grandkids, who (as we'll see) are shaping up (or rather, not shaping up) to be sedentary and overweight to an extent that's without precedent in human history. Such is their bulge, they look set to be placing demands on the health system themselves at precisely the moment their olds will be needing them to be furiously earning and paying taxes.

What's more, it's in the nature of modern medicine that healthcare gets progressively more expensive as it becomes more intensively technological. You just have to open a newspaper these days to read about a new breakthrough in the treatment of some disease or disorder or another: this, of course, is no coincidence, as newspapers are largely a medium of the baby boomers, and they're more than a little interested in hearing that the development of an elixir of youth is that much closer. Because of the way we've always done healthcare in this country, no sooner do we learn of a new treatment for what ails us than we demand it as of right. The consequence is that with every day that passes, those who make the decisions about where the health budget is spent are confronted by a wider range of treatments and procedures vying for our health dollar.

And worse is yet to come. Our health system has inevitably become more and more exposed to the global healthcare market, which dictates how much drugs cost and how much healthcare professionals get paid. World prices for both are going up, and will continue to go up, at a rate that will not be matched by our ability to pay.

As it stands, we simply won't be able to pay for everything we'll want out of the health system. Indeed – and although it only occasionally comes to public notice – we can't afford it now. While politicians on the Opposition benches raise a hue and cry whenever a government proposes any form of 'rationing' of health services, the provision of a public health system has always been a juggling act. Governments have always had to decide where to draw the line between what (and who) gets funded and who misses out on what. It's just that the line is set to shift dramatically in the very near future.

Thanks to the appetites of the baby boomers, there are countless self-help books out there on the subject of your health and what to do about it. Drink is bad for you, but red wine may be good for your heart. Coffee seems to ward off Alzheimer's, but it may cause liver cancer. Cholesterol is bad for you, but some of it is essential. Eat and drink less of some things, more of others, none of this, all of that. Give up smoking, take up jogging. Shun toxins. Seek out organics. Stay active, but avoid overdoing it. Stretch, meditate, exfoliate, rehydrate… we're not qualified to give you an opinion on the merits of these.

Instead, this book has been written in the same spirit as the earlier books on saving for retirement, Pension Panic, Kiwisafer and After the Panic. Because, after all, the principle is identical. When it comes to providing for a comfortable future, forewarned is forearmed. All that money you're salting away against your retirement will be little use to you if you don't have your health, or if you end up blowing it all on the pills, potions and procedures you reckon you need to get or stay well, rather than on your dream of spending your golden years motorcycling around the world.

As with the other three books, the approach taken here is to give you an idea of how policy is determined and how the healthcare scene will likely look by the time you find yourself wearing a track to your doctor's door. It's intended to help you make informed decisions not only as a consumer of healthcare services, but also as a citizen who is asked to judge the health policy offerings of rival political parties once every three years.

In Chapter One, we'll have a look at the history of our health system, partly for our entertainment, partly for our edification, and partly to understand how, as a nation, we devised the present system. After all, any physician worth their salt does their best to ascertain their patient's medical history before proceeding to a diagnosis and treatment.

In the next two chapters, we'll set about checking out the patients' vital signs. How adequately does the New Zealand healthcare system deliver? And what about that niggling pain, that worrying rash – the occasional scares and scandals that are splashed over the front pages and the six o'clock news? Are they the symptom of systemic disease? Will the system survive the looming winter of baby boomer discontent?

In Chapters Four and Five, we'll debunk the founding myth of New Zealand healthcare, namely that the public system can provide universal, comprehensive care for free and forever. A quick Health Warning here: we'll be talking about people's lives in terms of money, a concept that New Zealanders traditionally find repugnant. We'll show how 'prioritisation' – a gastric-coated word for rationing – is with us now, and is here to stay. We'll look at how prioritisation happens in the present system, and the pros and cons of the way it's done.

In the Chapters Six and Seven, we'll look to the future. What are the big trends that our health system will face? What do they mean for the way the system is structured and presently functions? And finally, we'll look at treatment options. What should we hope for from our healthcare system in the future, and what should we, as consumers of the services it delivers, do to ensure our own needs are met?

The question that motivated this book was simple. Is the New Zealand public health system outstanding, world's best practice, is it average or is it a crock? With the share of our collective income that we devote to health spending going up and predicted to go up a lot more yet, something seems amiss. Normally you would be determined to spend less on something once you had got your fill, yet the healthier we get the more we're determined to spend as we doggedly try to squeeze still more benefits from our health system. Clearly health isn't normal. Does this mean there's something wrong, or is health just different from other forms of commerce? This book seeks the answers to these questions.

Our approach to getting clarity on what makes our health sector tick and where its future lies has been to survey the literature on international comparisons of health systems, review what's been written specifically about the New Zealand health system, and finally and crucially conduct a series of interviews with health professionals operating within our system and get their perspectives of the positives and negatives of the system as it currently stands, considering their suggestions for improvement. That feedback from those who spend their days in the system has proved invaluable in getting to grips with what the major issues are – whether they be doctors, nurses, administrators or patients. A summary of the feedback from those interviews is provided on the website that's associated with the book, www.healthcheque.co.nz.

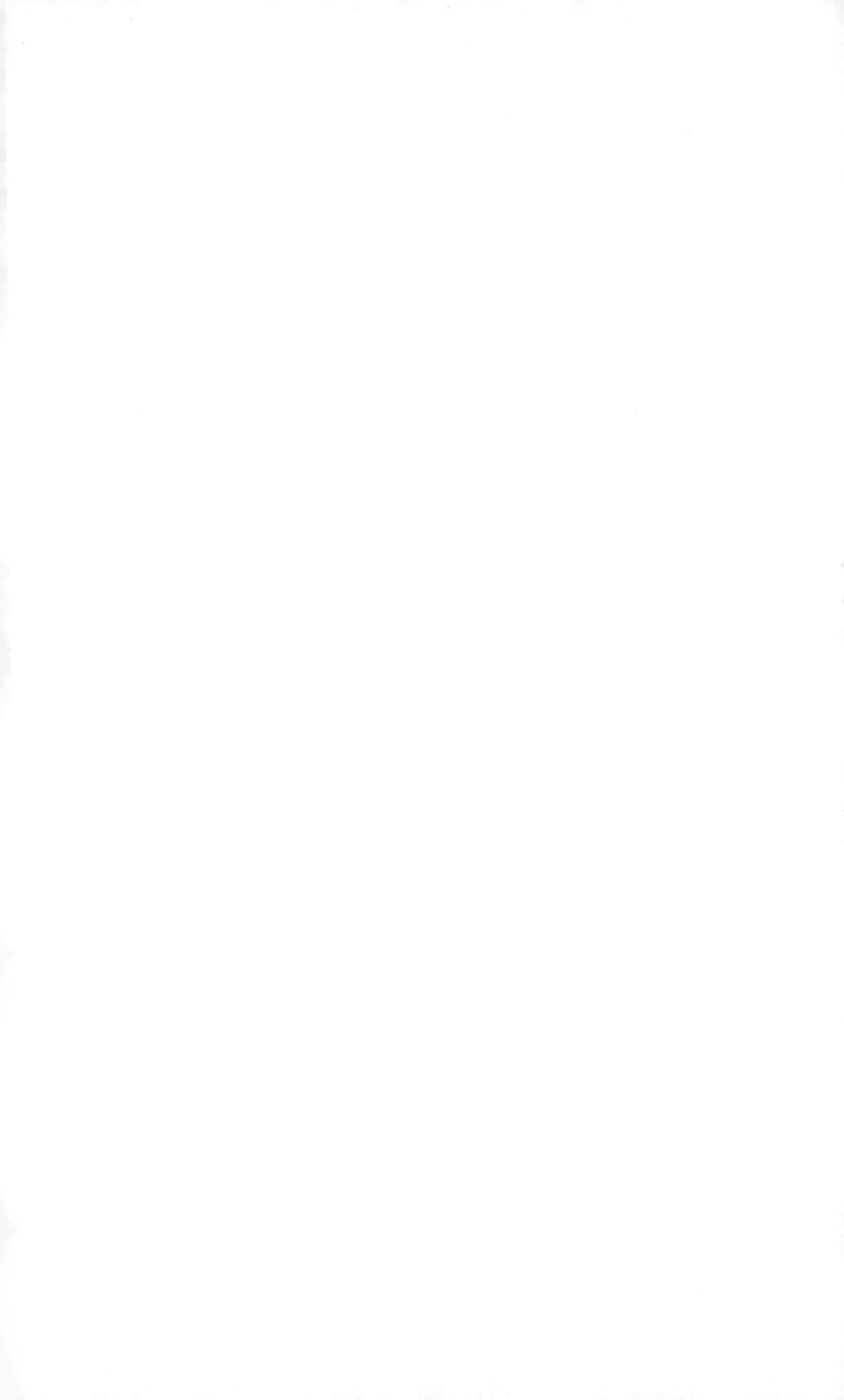

Chapter 1

EVOLUTION AND REVOLU+ION[1]

One of the very first questions that arises in relation to any public health system is: why is the government involved in the provision of health services at all? Surely a body's health is his or her own responsibility and concern. Why should taxes be levied on society in order to make health services available to individuals, rather than simply encouraging individuals to take prudent steps to ensure they can purchase the necessary services as required? It's a valid question. After all, the Americans earnestly believe it's nuts to make wealthy citizens underwrite the health of the down-at-heel as well as their own.

Market failure in healthcare – the foundation of New Zealand's approach

This whole book could be about whether the Government should provide healthcare or whether we should pay for it ourselves, whether the US system – with its gold-plated facilities for some, bog-basic health services for others and even denial of access for some of its citizens – is a better approach than our universal entitlement and mix of State and Private delivered health services. In different countries there seem to be plenty of different ways to skin a cat when it comes to funding and providing healthcare. All different systems have their pros and cons, and all-in-all, we don't think it is worth the upheaval of changing our system entirely. In case you are interested, here are a few reasons why:

1. Healthcare investments are big and specialised. In a country of our size this can make it hard to have a truly competitive market.

2. Docs know more about our health than we do, so we are at their mercy when it comes to providing treatment. Will they act in our

interest? If docs over-treat us, would we know? As Abraham Maslow said *'He that is good with a hammer tends to think everything is a nail.'* This imbalance of power gets even worse in the emergency room. This is known as supplier-induced demand.

3. If you can afford to pay for treatment, it's odds-on that you don't need it. In a completely free market system the rich do tend to stay healthy and the sick stay poor – even with insurance. This disparity doesn't scream for changing the New Zealand approach.

4. If by some miracle insurance was the answer, you'd have little reason to look after yourself. Ever wondered why Kiwis play rugby and invented bungy jumping? Because ACC reduces the risk!

5. One person's health sometimes affects another, for example with contagious diseases. That is the historical origin of State intervention in healthcare, particularly through inoculation and public health programmes.

6. As with pensions, people can't or don't think far enough ahead, and so left to their own devices they under-invest in prevention. That myopia ultimately drives up their health costs.

We could go on, but there isn't much point. Suffice to say this book will focus on the issues around getting our current system working better, rather than dreaming up a whizz-bang new healthcare system.

In order to understand the answer – and why in New Zealand the question has been so earnestly posed again over the last 20 years – it helps to have a bit of a look at the evolution of modern medicine, and of the way in which our medical services have been arranged over the last 170 years.

A stroll down medical memory lane is like a visit to a fairground house of horrors. Before the rise of modern science which, for these purposes, is little more than 150 years old, medicine was based on a mixture of folklore, badly mistaken beliefs and even more woefully misguided wisdom. A visitor to early modern Europe would find little they recognised amongst the available health providers back then (unless, of course, that visitor was a loyal customer of modern 'alternative' therapy): physicians, for the most part, believed that health consisted of the balance of four vital fluids in the body (the 'four humours'), which were influenced by diet, exercise and moral character. Disease, on the other hand, occurred where the humours were out of whack, and while this imbalance could occasionally be treated by relatively non-invasive means – by including certain medicinal herbs or potions in your diet, say, changing your exercise regimen or mending your sinful ways – the most popular method was blood-letting. A vein or an artery was opened and blood allowed to flow until you passed out, which was taken to be a sign the treatment was working. Sometimes, a physician would prescribe a course of leeches to achieve the desired blood loss – European medicine offered the high life to hundreds of millions of these slimy little critters in the eighteenth century alone – but mostly, the method was to cut a blood vessel, and until the middle of the eighteenth century, the person who carried out the procedure was the same bloke who cut your hair when you were in the pink of health. For it's often overlooked in today's set-up that the highly-paid, Porsche-driving, golf-addicted, beachfront property-owning chap who gently chides you for calling him 'Doctor' ('Ahem. It's Mister'.) as he breezes in and tells you which bits of you he's going to carve up is enjoying a social status that his profession has only come to enjoy in the last few decades. As late as 1745, British surgeons belonged to an organisation named the Company of Barber-Surgeons, consisting of those people whom you trusted enough to use sharp things on your person when need arose (when you needed a shave, for example, a fringe trim or simply a gangrenous limb amputated). Interestingly, the red-and-white striped pole that barbers still display symbolises the blood and the bandages, but you'd have to reckon barbers would trade the insignia for the salary commanded today by that breakaway branch of their venerable guild.

Further back, of course, medicine just gets grislier. Since the time of the ancients, there was always a class of person about who was willing to have a crack at setting your broken bones for you, or boring a hole in your skull to let the evil spirits out (a process called trepanning), or bringing your child into the world by Caesarean section (which was seldom, if ever, survivable by the mother until the principles of wound management and the causes of infection began to be understood in the twentieth century). But thankfully, we have no need to go there.

When James Cook sailed from Blighty bound for the Pacific and his historic rendezvous with these happy isles in 1769, he left an England that possessed nothing resembling a 'public health system'. There were hospitals, but these were set up at the bequest of wealthy individuals to provide the dubious benefits of eighteenth century medicine to the poor. Private individuals shifted for themselves, seeking to self-cure, or consulting physicians or surgeons (or herbalists, or apothecaries, or witches, or who knows, but probably barbers, too) who were private businesspeople. Since medical treatment was broadly ineffective, it wasn't much of a private commodity, let alone one demanded as a public good by the majority of the population. The standard approach to preventive medicine was to pray: pray for the health of yourself and others.

Little had changed by the time New Zealand came to be settled – or at least, little in England. In New Zealand, of course, a huge proportion of the Maori hadn't survived their first exposure to diseases that caused a mere sniffle in Europeans, who had built up an immunity over the centuries. In the absence of any inkling of epidemiology, European visitors to new lands watched the locals keeling over like ninepins and put it all down to the major cause of misfortune, disease and unexplained death in that paradigm, namely the Lord with His nose out of joint. The logic of the argument that ran: *'We stay well because we love and worship Jesus Christ. You sicken and die because you're a silly pagan and don't.'* proved seductive, and accounts for much of the rapid traction that Christianity was able to gain amongst afflicted indigenous populations after first contact.

But the century after the signing of the Treaty of Waitangi saw medicine revolutionised, as science began to make real inroads into the causes of disease. The theory of the four humours began to fall out of favour, doubtless spelling disaster for leech-breeding enterprises (although you could still find the odd sawbones swearing by a nice bleed well into the twentieth century). The work of Louis Pasteur and others suggested that microscopic organisms might have something to do with quite a lot of illness. Over time doctors jettisoned their bizarre treatments and became experts at diagnosis, but as yet they had few remedies other than good food, clean water and fresh air. Pasteur and Robert Koch also realised that the various tribes of microbes were constantly at war with one another, and that one might be enlisted in the fight against another – the principle of antibiotics. The first synthetic antibiotic, Salversen, was produced in the 1880s (although it was nearly as bad for you as the majority of the diseases it was competent to treat). Other, more congenial versions were soon to follow.

The plaster-of-Paris cast to set and immobilise fractures was developed in 1851 (although the principle of winding around a broken limb bandages soaked in a fluid that would subsequently harden had been known in the Middle Ages, where battlefield injuries were often swathed in cloth soaked in horses' blood, of which there was no shortage on Mediæval battlefields). Someone had the guts to attempt surgery on the heart of a living patient as early as the 1890s, and the first cornea transplant was successfully performed in 1905. Both are remarkable when it's considered that most of the more effective anaesthetics – morphine, ether and cocaine – were still mostly regarded as recreational drugs at upper class parties rather than of any use in surgery, and it wasn't until the 1950s that your anaesthetist could look you in the eye and give you better-than-even odds that you'd wake up from a general.

World War I worked wonders on trauma surgery, even if it's one of the tragedies of history that hundreds of thousands of lives would doubtless have been saved if the first truly effective antibiotic, penicillin, had been discovered just a decade earlier (it was discovered in 1925). But it is to the so-called Spanish Flu pandemic of 1918 that New Zealanders really owe their national public health system. When the virus was in full swing here, busily carrying away an estimated 6,716 lives (5,516 of them Maori), it showed up the inadequacies of the existing, fragmented system at precisely the moment in history when it became possible to imagine an alternative.

At the turn of the nineteenth and twentieth centuries, arranging for medical treatment for an illness or an injury was overwhelmingly a private affair. You felt sick, you took yourself off to your doctor, or had him visit at home (as some old-timers still remember doctors being prepared to do). Most healthcare was administered in New Zealand by general practitioners, a surprising disproportion of who had studied at Edinburgh University, which boasted the United Kingdom's top medical school. The family doctor occupied a revered position in New Zealand society, and they were rewarded commensurately: an indicator of their relative status is that when motorcars first began to proliferate on our roads after about 1905, it was overwhelmingly doctors who owned them. Not only did motorcars help in making house-calls (no more tiresome catching and harnessing that bloody horse), but they were fiendishly expensive, costing roughly three times the annual average wage.

The first hospitals in this country were established at the behest of Governor George Grey, who decreed in 1847 that facilities should be built in Auckland, New Plymouth, Wellington and Wanganui and made available to Maori as well as Pakeha. Provincial government got in on the act with the establishment of 'Charitable Aid and Hospital Boards' – as the name suggests, hospital care was mostly targeted at the poor and Maori as part of municipal charity – and while these received some funding from the Colonial administration, central government didn't assume their responsibilities when the provinces were abolished in 1875. The provision of hospitals was presumed to be a local responsibility; the main centres had all established Charitable Aid and Hospital Boards of their own by the mid-1880s. Not, of course, that the hospitals did the poor or Maori or anyone, for that matter, much real good: their main function was to quarantine sufferers of the epidemics that periodically broke out. Some even specialised in particular diseases, such as the leper's colony on Quail Island in Lyttleton Harbour until 1920, or the various sanatoria that were established for sufferers of tuberculosis in the early years of the twentieth century.

Of far more significance than the early Hospital Boards were the various Health Boards set up by local government under the Public Health Act of 1872. The twenty-first century Kiwi will naturally presume that these were charged with providing medical services, but in fact, they undertook works designed to improve the sanitary conditions of their respective areas – drainage and the control of effluent, keeping livestock and their exhaust away from people and their dwellings, removing and disposing of the dead (human and animal) in a timely, efficient and hygienic manner – and these measures were incalculably more effective in maintaining the health of the general population than all the hospitals and all the doctors and nurses were in restoring it. Bacterial diseases such as typhoid fever were as much of a scourge in 1870s Christchurch, for example, as boy racers are today. Built on a swamp and with nowhere much for sewage to run to, the Garden City then had the reputation as New Zealand's unhealthiest town, with twice the national mortality rate. But the Christchurch Health Board – established as a department of the Drainage Board – mounted a concerted campaign to replace cesspits with nightsoil collection, and the results were dramatic: less sewage in the artesian drinking water meant fewer typhoid outbreaks, and fewer Christchurch residents banging on the pearly gates.[2]

In fact, though, the Health Boards (Christchurch excepted) were rather lethargic in the discharge of their duties until an outbreak of bubonic plague in Australia in 1900 focused everyone's attention on hygiene. Soon after New Zealand reported its first (and only) case, the government passed a new Public Health Act, which made the prevention of disease and the conditions that gave rise to it a national responsibility. A further measure to secure this end was taken in 1909, when the Public Health Department assumed administration of the nation's hospitals, or at least, those belonging to local bodies.

As we've noted, whereas we understand the term 'public health system' to refer to doctors, nurses and hospitals busily curing people of their ills and rewarded for it out of the state coffers, our great-great-grandparents had a different understanding. Public health was all about prevention. The first impetus toward coordinating and nationalising health services came from this kind of focus on prevention. Healthcare was a public good, that is, because as the plague scare, a smallpox epidemic in 1913 (which predictably hit Maori far harder than Pakeha) and then the Spanish Flu made clear, an individual's private health woes can swiftly become everyone's problem.

By the 1920s, however, medical care was also becoming something worth having. The range of diseases, disorders and disasters it could address and even ameliorate was widening, and for the first time, the dream of healthcare as a public good – to be made available to all and funded out of the tax take – began to be dreamed. Although it was on the agenda in the 1920s, it wasn't until the advent of the First Labour Government that things started to move on nationalisation. Perhaps this was because most aspects of devil-take-the-hindmost capitalism, including private healthcare provision, had lately been discredited in the Great Depression, and the populace was in the mood for a new model. Amongst their measures designed to ensure the 'cradle to grave' welfare of New Zealanders, Michael Joseph Savage and his Cabinet proposed a universal healthcare system that would be free at the point of use, giving all New Zealanders access to quality healthcare in a timely fashion. The medical staff of state-owned hospitals would be paid salaries, so their income wouldn't depend on the number of treatments given. This was calculated to create a focus on prevention of disease rather than its treatment: naturally, if your cash register rings every time a patient walks through the door, you'll be anxious to see them as often as possible and you won't be too insistent that they wash their hands every time they go to the toilet. It creates an incentive, that is, to under-prevent and over-treat.

Labour's plans were mostly executed in 1938 – 'mostly', because it was a radical suite of reforms, and proved frankly too Marxist by far for general practitioners, who were private businesspeople after all and wanted to retain that freedom. The GPs demanded the right to work in either the private or public sectors (or both), and to charge patients who could afford it as they saw fit and as the market would bear. The government was forced to play ball, and offered a subsidy of around two-thirds for visits to the family doctor. Nationalisation thus only really applied to about 80-85% of what we'll now start to call the 'secondary health system' (hospital beds) and apart from the subsidy, left GPs – the backbone of the 'primary system' – untouched. The poor (especially Maori) still struggled to access care, and the hoped-for incentive to minimise illnesses in the general population never materialised. Nor did Savage and Peter Fraser, his Minister of Health, get dental care included, as they'd hoped.

Even if it was only a partial success, it was a bold plan, conceived at the dawn of modern scientific medicine. It couldn't have been imagined much earlier – as we've noted, there wasn't much in the way of effective medical treatment to nationalise – and if it had been left too much later, it might have appeared simply impossible, as it always has to the United States. After all, this was just the beginning of the dizzying efflorescence of drugs and procedures that continues to this day. It may have appeared to Savage and his advisers in the mid-1930s that there was a finite range of effective treatments available to distribute and that centralised distribution would be more efficient, as some historians assert.[3] Ten years later, at the end of World War II, the repertoire of medical science's wizardry had increased exponentially, and the pace was picking up. Promising to fully fund every treatment for all would have seemed like a bit of a pipe dream, even then.

Nonetheless, the major and lasting achievement of Savage's plan was to create precisely this expectation in New Zealanders, who (apart from GPs) pretty much universally approved of it. A sacred cow had been born, and it's this expectation that has dogged all subsequent attempts both to fund and to reform the health system, as we shall see.

The subsequent history of New Zealand's health system (as established by the First Labour Government in the 1930s) has been described as consisting of an *evolutionary* phase, giving way to a more recent *revolutionary* phase. Nothing much changed in the evolutionary phase. For the next 50 years, until the late 1980s, there were 30 Hospital Boards varying in size from Auckland to the tiny Maniototo, which served a piffling 2600 people. Each hospital was led by a management team: the chief administrator controlled all 26 administrative requirements (e.g., buildings, cleaning, finances), the matron/chief nurse controlled all nursing staff and the medical superintendent had oversight of the medical staff. None of the team had overall decision-making power, although anecdotally, on the accounts of those personally scarred by the experience, one personality tended to dominate. This team reported to the Hospital Board, which was made up of elected representatives and members of the community that the hospital served.

To anyone familiar with the complexity of modern hospital administration, it doesn't look like a very sophisticated structure: one doc, one nurse and one bean-counter for each hospital. In reality, there were probably a few helpers in the mix, but the formal requirements were little more exacting than this. The system didn't generate a lot of paperwork, and no one really stood on the niceties of managerial procedures or processes. These features could be seen as a virtue. But nor did it produce a lot of information on which we can now judge the system's performance. Before we get too carried away with this shortcoming, however, it's worth pointing out – as we'll see later – that all the reforms and upheavals of recent decades haven't yielded much in the way of solid performance information, either, or at least nothing that can convince you there's been a dramatic improvement. The capacity of modern hospital administration to produce paperwork is phenomenal; the usefulness of all that information in gauging the performance of hospitals is rather less impressive.

While the wheels stayed on the machine and things kept ticking over without the raft of administrators we need today, reform was talked about frequently enough. The most popular topics, for those brave enough to raise them, were boundary changes for Hospital Board catchments, or bringing the GPs and the hospitals closer together. The GPs were as averse as ever to any kind of change that offended their entrepreneurial instincts, and the public were on the alert for anything that might mean they would lose their local hospital. In fact, the only major change to our health system before the 1980s was the creation of the Accident Compensation Corporation (ACC) in 1975.

ACC is unique in the world, and was set up to prevent the need for suing over accidents. New Zealanders sacrificed their right to sue, and instead got a 'no fault' social insurance system (the premiums for this insurance are compulsory: you cannot opt out). This grants an accident victim both the right to a suite of rehabilitative treatment, and to compensation for loss of income or permanent disability. ACC is funded by various levies, such as the Earner's Premium, which currently lifts around 1.7 cents of every dollar in your pay-packet, and the Employer Premium, which intercepts a further 1.3 cents before it even reaches your pay-packet. The rationale is that the earner insures themselves for the risky behaviour they indulge in outside work (playing rugby, picking fights with heavy dudes at the boozer) and the employer insures against the dangers of the workplace. There's also a significant ACC levy built into the cost of petrol at the pump and into your motor vehicle registration fees to pick up some of the health bill occasioned by the way we drive our cars. If the cost of providing ACC goes up, the levies automatically follow so that the budget grows to match the increased cost. One of the first unpleasant duties John Key was obliged to discharge as prime minister was to announce that precisely this was just about to happen. According to the most recent figures, ACC's current liabilities (existing claims on which it is obliged to pay out) amount to \$23.8 billion, compared with assets of just \$11 billion.[4] The government claims that the scheme's very viability is now in doubt.

Under ACC, you're not only assured treatment, but if you're employed, ACC have a positive incentive to treat you as soon as possible. ACC pays 80% of your salary if you're injured, so the sooner they get you fit and healthy and generating levies again, the better for them. The incentive seems to work. You don't hear of ACC patients languishing on a waiting list for six months. It's a different story if you have a health problem that is not accident-related. If you lose your mobility or your income through such a misfortune, you're pretty much on your own: no one is obliged to compensate you, and the best you can hope for is a sickness benefit from Social Welfare. Your treatment is at the discretion of the public healthcare system. You don't have an automatic right to treatment, nor any assurance over what treatments are available year to year (as some social insurance schemes in other parts of the world provide). The budget is fixed, so in theory and regardless of your earning power or status or prospects in society, your needs are weighed against those of others waiting for care.

Anomalies between the treatment of accident and illness victims abound, and are perhaps at their starkest in cases of those with lifelong disability, such as in the case study below.

The Handley family[5]

During the birth of her second child Daniel, Sharon Handley experienced severe complications. Daniel should have been delivered via caesarean section, instead he had to be resuscitated for nine and a half minutes before taking his first breath. Daniel was expected to be a vegetable. Incredibly, he emerged from the ordeal with his senses and sensibilities intact, however, albeit with severe cerebral palsy and spastic quadriplegia.

Despite having all his faculties, Daniel needs constant care to survive. The risk that he will choke to death is ever-present. Sharon had dedicated herself to caring for Daniel for the first five years of his life before they were told that Daniel might be eligible for an ACC claim. Even though Daniel never had an income to replace (ACC replaces up to 80% of your pre injury income), the difference between the care he was getting and what he could get if ACC became involved was stark.

If Daniel's misadventure was deemed to be an injury, he would be entitled to round-the-clock care, and the caregiver (Sharon) could be paid for her role. If, on the other hand, it were deemed an 'illness', ACC wouldn't touch his case. Rather, as an illness beneficiary he would be means-tested before any care was offered and the maximum amount of care would be capped at 30 hours per week.

What's more, injury victims are entitled to an array of capital improvements and modifications to their houses and their cars, and to all disability and medical equipment that may help the condition. Once again, illness victims' entitlements are means-tested and capped at very low levels. A car modified for disability often costs over $110,000. Injury victims get the car for free; illness victims get just $24,000[6] toward the cost. Incredibly, illness victims who are disabled are ineligible for mobility equipment other than what they need to get around inside their own home. The healthcare system is clearly happy to see illness victims under house arrest: your home is your castle, but you'd prefer to have the key.

Back to the case. It wasn't immediately clear to ACC that Daniel was the victim of an injury. They thought it looked like an illness. After five years of legal battles and table thumping, the kindly Corporation finally stumped up for all Daniel's care – backdated. But for every good news story, there's another disabled person who doesn't quite qualify as an injury victim, and is left to the mercy of the Corporation's poor cousin – the public healthcare system.

Four years ago Sasha (aged 12) was riding her bike to school when she suddenly felt dizzy. Sensibly, she got off her bike, and promptly suffered a major stroke. Sasha was left severely disabled, and her mother had to give up work to look after her. And it was her further bad luck to have suffered this affliction as the result of an illness. Had an accident been the cause of the disability, Sasha's mother would have been paid to look after her. As it was, Sasha and her mother receive only the minimal assistance available through Social Welfare and the Ministry of Health. The moral of the story? If you come over all funny as you're pedalling along, pick the nearest power pole and crash into it.[7]

The rationale for ACC is that the country saves money by virtually eliminating lawsuits arising from accidents and injuries. And it's a convenient spin-off that denying a whole raft of people the same level of entitlement available to the victims of accidents saves the country even more. None of it makes the anomalies look any better.

With the addition of ACC, New Zealand was left with a health system that was quite unusual internationally. There were, in effect, three parallel health systems. It had a tax-funded public system, another that was funded directly by users or their private insurers, and a compulsory and universal 'social insurance' scheme (ACC) funded from direct levies (a tax by any other name).

Health under the knife –
the Lange/Douglas/Bassett razor gang

Just as the Savage government secured a mandate for radical change from a population left despondent and hungry for change by the Great Depression, the fourth Labour Government that was installed in 1984 considered itself to be under strict instructions from the electorate to do pretty much anything but what Rob Muldoon had been doing for the past decade. For the electorate, of course, it proved to be very much a case of 'be careful what you wish for', as the Labour government proceeded to slash, burn and privatise all manner of aspects of state and society under the nice, friendly umbrella term, 'reform'. Compared to some areas, health got off lightly – for the time being.

In fact, as with much of what the fourth Labour Government likes to claim as its very own work, the ideas it put into practice in health in the 1980s had been around in the bureaucracy for as much as a decade. The problem of fragmentation and duplication in the health system had been identified in a White Paper to Norman Kirk's third Labour Government in 1974, and Muldoon himself had tinkered with some of its suggestions. With a freer hand than its predecessors, Lange's government embraced the proposed 'reforms' with gusto. The 30 Hospital Boards were reorganised into 14 Area Health Boards (AHBs), whose responsibilities were extended from simply running the hospitals to planning the health of the local population (in a sense that recalled the preventive focus of the Public Health

Department of a century earlier). In other words, they now had to plan prevention and primary care as well as deliver the secondary system. The funding formula was also changed, from one based on divvying up the budget according to a formula derived from historical proportions to one based on population numbers, with some tweaking permissible to take account of populations with peculiarly high need (notably those featuring Maori and Pacific Island communities). However, there were teething problems with this: the AHBs were in various states of financial health, and like most other workers in New Zealand, health sector employees were starting to demand wage rises after many years of stagnation, spiralling inflation and even a wage freeze.

The Boards of the AHBs still comprised two-thirds of members who were locally elected, but the remaining third were now directly appointed by the Minister of Health. The AHB model put a much greater emphasis on efficiency and accountability to the Government. In line with the broad thrust of Labour's public sector reform, more 'business-like' management structures were put in place, and goals and targets were set according to which the performance of an AHB was supposed to be judged.

Who cut the CHEs? –
National's competitive business model for public health

While they were generously given a second term, just in case all the pain they were inflicting was for some worthwhile purpose after all, the appalled electorate booted Labour out in 1990. Imagine their surprise when the National government assembled by Jim Bolger began scouring the landscape for anything green that might have survived the scorched-earth years under Rogernomics. The property and stockmarkets had crashed in 1987, and recessionary gloom had settled over the land. That didn't stop costs rising in the health portfolio.

Health was in for it this time. Labour had assembled a taskforce under businessman Alan Gibbs that was charged with finding ways of cutting costs and improving efficiency in the health sector, and the result was a report that emerged in 1988 ominously entitled 'Unshackling the Hospitals'. The new National Health Minister Simon Upton then worked the ideas up into an action plan. The plan was twofold: to focus public funding on the most important treatments and the neediest patients, and to improve the efficiency of the hospital system. Gibbs boldly proclaimed that substantial productivity gains would be captured if hospitals were run along business lines, although he was fuzzy about what that actually meant. It seemed that the ultimate objective would be privatisation of delivery – that is, hospitals would be privately owned (or at least, run as though they were) and would compete for funding supplied by the government. This unleashing of competition would turn hospitals into lean, mean treatment machines.

Even the easy bit proved harder than Gibbs (and National) expected. The starting point was that New Zealand should be able to define a set of services to which everyone was entitled, to be called 'Core Health Services'. Another taskforce was set up, and began consulting with communities all around the country and trying to fit their hopes, dreams and aspirations into the template, namely an American list of such services called 'the Oregon list'. This runs to 93 pages of small type, and – surprise, surprise – everyone wanted every little nip, tuck, potion and pill listed there, and more besides, and they wanted them for free. It was that Banquo's ghost, the shade of Mickey Savage, smiling benignly at the table: the ingrained expectation of universal and comprehensive healthcare, forever and ever, world without end, amen.

Consultation put the government in the awkward position of the parent who must tell their child that there's no such person as Santa. Rationing of health services was not only a real and present threat that the nation faced: health professionals had been doing it for years. So the sensible debate over what services we could and should provide for ourselves was sidelined for the futile debate over whether there should be rationing at all. The media loved it, and we were treated to the first of what has become a whole genre of news story: the hapless, faithfully taxpaying Kiwi condemned to die by heartless bureaucrats because the lifesaving treatment s/he needs is deemed too expensive. In this case, the unlucky one was Rau Williams, whose story we repeat below for the benefit of anyone who was under a rock in the late 1990s.

Rau Williams

Rau was a 63-year-old Maori man with diabetes and moderate dementia who was experiencing end-stage renal failure (his kidneys had packed up). After making a detailed assessment, the hospital decided to discontinue treatment. Dialysis is expensive – it costs between $30,000 and $80,000 per year, per patient.[8] Rau couldn't do the dialysis unsupervised because of his dementia, so the cost would have been at the upper end of that scale. Regional Health Authority guidelines at the time stated that to justify this spending, two extra years of life would be needed. Rau was expected to live a year if he was lucky.

The decision to discontinue treatment was legally challenged by Rau's family, and the case drew considerable media attention. It was argued that Rau didn't want to die and that his doctors had a duty to treat him. The Courts didn't agree, and the decision to withdraw treatment was upheld. Sadly but inevitably, Rau died on 10 October 1997.

The courts were uneasy that doctors slavishly following guidelines could in effect sentence a man to death, but it was decided that as long as the guidelines simply guided the doctors' decision, it was conscionable under the brand new Human Rights Act. Curiously and incredibly, the judgements in this case never drew attention to the fact that prioritising of resources was routine and widespread in the New Zealand health system. A golden opportunity to stand behind the doctors in some of the tough decisions that they have to make in prioritising end-of-life treatment was thus lost.[9]

Decisions like those made in the Rau Williams case are never easy for doctors, patients, their families or the public. No-one deserves to die when the medical means to prevent their death are available, but neither do we have unlimited resources. Given our ageing population, and the rise of diabetes, patients like Rau have the potential to overwhelm our health system. For every Rau Williams kept alive for another couple of (probably unproductive) years, a younger person, with a more extensive future ahead of them, is deprived.

The second reform – and, in fact, the most successful – of the measures introduced by National in the 1990s was the creation of the state drug-buying agency, Pharmac. Prioritisation was the whole raison d'être of Pharmac: in order to reduce budget blowouts on drugs, National appointed a body to oversee the pharmaceutical budget and work out where the biggest bang for the tax buck could be had – the maximum therapeutic benefit to patients for each dollar spent, based on the best available evidence. Based on its determinations, Pharmac gives doctors an approved list of drugs from which they can prescribe with a public subsidy. Anything else you want, you have to buy yourself.

Pharmac's approach also yields the advantage of bulk buying power, which enables it to 'shake down' the giant drug companies, securing further savings for the New Zealand taxpayer. It seems a simple model, really, and so effective that the US government keeps insisting, on behalf of the giant, rapacious American drug companies, that New Zealand abolish it as a necessary precondition for any free trade deal. Yet it hadn't been tried here before National was bold enough to give it a whirl, and few organisations like it exist in the world. Pity the National government was elected in 2008 on a promise to undermine it, and has proved as good as its word. More on this shortly.

Later in life, Alan Gibbs would become famous for designing an amphibious car that actually goes as well on water as it does on land. But when National drove the third big idea contained within the Gibbs Report down the boat-ramp, it just kept going with all hands, until greasy little bubbles were about all that could be seen.

The third big idea of the 1990-1999 National Government was the purchaser/provider split. By comparing different hospitals, it was noticed that there was a difference of about one third in the cost per procedure. The difference, it was presumed, arose from efficiency. It was felt that if each hospital became as efficient as the most efficient one, the country could have more operations for the same outlay. So what stops a hospital from being efficient? Why, it's the lack of competition, of course! Without competition, there's nothing to fear, or aspire to beat. If the same people in charge of dishing out the money locally also ran the hospital, there was no hope of introducing competitive pressures, either. So if your 'silver bullet' solution to inefficiencies in the public sector health system is to make hospitals 'compete', then clearly a revolution in the way the whole funding system operated was required. And it came. The National Government set up hospitals to run like businesses, competing for the right to cut you up, and the key to getting them to compete was to separate the *purchasing* and *providing* functions of hospitals.

Under the pre-existing scheme, AHBs were responsible not only for the hospitals they ran, but for the health of the general population in their area as well. But it was plain that the general health of the population took a back seat to the interests of their hospitals when it came to doling out the money. There was no way they would pay another hospital to do an operation for patients from their area if there was any way their own hospital could treat them, regardless of whether other hospitals could offer them better or even more effective treatment. AHBs lived and died by keeping their own hospitals running.

So National's big idea was to take the purchasing role off

AHBs, and vest it instead in four new Regional Health Authorities (RHAs). In effect, these were charged with purchasing the best and most effective treatment for the public from whichever hospital was best able to provide it. National was also going to allow people to take their allocated share of public funding and go to private insurers as well, but they canned this idea when they realised that private insurers would take all the rich, low-risk clients and the public sector would be left with all the basket cases. The 14 AHBs became 23 Crown Health Enterprises (CHEs), and they earned their money by competing against each other for the right to do operations funded by the RHAs. This competition, so the theory went, would force CHEs to improve quality and reduce costs or face going under.

It's a neat idea in theory.

Unfortunately it was all a little different in practice. Hospitals probably did get more efficient, but it turns out that efficiency isn't all we really want from a hospital. For one thing, efficiency doesn't take into account the quality of the procedures – an appendectomy executed at breakneck speed looks really efficient until the patient is readmitted a few days later with peritonitis. Nor does it take account of the relative levels of need of different patients. If you had to reduce the cost per hip replacement operation, you'd probably start by doing the easiest ones – nice, young, fit, skinny patients – rather than helping those who needed it most. It would be efficient, because you'd have replaced lots of hips without forking out too much money. But it would not be a fair approach to the cases of individuals whose need was greater, and the nation would be left with a whole hobbling cohort whose needs were not being met.

Trying to turn hospitals into businesses proved to be something you couldn't achieve overnight, too. To achieve the necessary cultural revolution, a fresh batch of suited and booted 'consultants' and career administrators were brought in from outside the health sector. With expertise in everything from manufacturing to software development, it was expected that the newcomers would inculcate hospital administration with fresh 'business thinking' and that they'd be free of the bias that arises from existing relationships with medical staff. Doctors disrespectfully refused to genuflect to the whizz-kids, and in cases where, say, an accomplished advertising executive tried to take responsibility for telling doctors what their ethical and clinical priorities should be, the level of dysfunction skyrocketed. One consultant interviewed by the Listener breezily admitted that he didn't know the difference between intensive care and post-operative recovery, but vowed he would find 20% in efficiency savings nonetheless.[10] Many senior managers left the system in disgust, and many staff and management who remained felt alienated and frustrated. The Health and Disability Commissioner's review of Gisborne Hospital, for example, found the organisation to be *'traumatised, unhappy, marked by suspicion and distrust.'* After three years, only three of the first flush of 23 new Chief Executives were still in their jobs, so the experiment with 'fresh thinking' clearly failed.

Further problems duly emerged. National's 'business model' eroded the effectiveness of cooperation amongst hospitals, and thus undermined the entire concept of a 'national health system'. CHEs stopped sharing innovations and information, as under the Commerce Act, this would have been seen as collusion. Now *that* was regulation gone nuts! In one fell swoop, by declaring hospitals to be commercial entities, the ability of all communities to benefit from an innovation made by one hospital was outlawed.

Hospitals also pulled back from their links with primary care, leaving GPs to spend most of the 1990s lost in the wilderness. But the crowning disgrace was the intractable problem of what to do with hospitals that failed to meet performance criteria. In the business world, failing businesses close. But no such discipline was applied here, for the simple reason that to shut down hospitals is political suicide. The public was already suspicious of the changes – we've already seen how explicit prioritisation raised the hackles of the media and public. What's more, the purchaser-provider split looked too much like a step toward privatisation and/or the closure of hospitals for most people's tastes. When, in the early days of its programme of reforms, National attempted to introduce part charges for hospital care, there was outrage at first, with many people simply refusing to pay. Jeers greeted the news when it became known that administrating the regime cost far more than was collected in fees. Poorly performing CHEs got bailed out, and good ones had their funding cut to pay for the bailouts. Little surprise, then, that in their first year, CHEs ran a combined deficit of almost $190m. The reorganisation had cost an estimated $270 million, as new agencies had to be set up and all those expensive consultants had to be lured across with the promise of fat fees. Consequently, the reforms never managed to generate anywhere close to the promised 20% productivity gain. There were improvements in efficiency, but it can be argued that these were simply a continuation of the trend started under AHBs. So after all the upheaval, CHEs were still swimming in red ink. The reforms hadn't even achieved their primary aim, economic efficiency.

Meanwhile, nothing about the realities of running a national health system had changed. The re-jigged system was just as pinched between the rock of limited resources and the hard place of increasing demand as its predecessors had been. Waiting lists continued to grow – from 64,000 in 1993 to over 94,000 in 1996. This meant one in forty people nationwide was waiting for an operation. When the internal spats between administrators and medical staff boiled over into public view, and highly visible problems arose – such as infections spreading through overcrowded wards – the writing was on the wall for the reforms.

National's 'competitive model' for the health sector was a sick ideological joke. No other country has experimented so recklessly with private sector models in a public sector health system – and now we know why. Patently, the reforms were fundamentally flawed, not least because they couldn't be followed through. The analysis of how the whole thing would work was simply too shallow. Yes, there were efficiency disparities between hospitals, but the dead-eyed ideologue's fancy that competition could sort out hospitals as readily as it did pizza delivery concerns had zero analytical foundation, completely ignoring the full gambit of what the public requires from its health system. Its rapid failure was proof of that. National hadn't equipped itself with any way of measuring, judging or proving the success of the reforms, but it's hard to find measures that show what happened in a positive light. Of course, you'll still find a hack or two who claim the reforms didn't work because they weren't implemented right and too many compromises were made.[11] But to most, this era will remain a timely reminder that massive reforms need to be carefully considered, and that excluding the staff who work in the target area is a risky tactic.

Naturally, National's bold package of reforms was slowly wound back by the National/ NZ First coalition that succeeded it in office in 1996. The four purchasers of healthcare, the Regional Health Authorities, were combined into one national purchaser – the Health Funding Authority (HFA). The changes shifted the ethos from competition to working collaboratively with staff, better performance management and clearer prioritisation of resources. Many health sector people we interviewed for this project felt that this last permutation of the 1990s reforms was probably the best arrangement New Zealand has ever had. Tragically, it was too good to last. The model was just starting to bed down when the Labour/Alliance Government was elected in 1999 and lifted the bonnet all over again.

Something for everyone...

The incoming Labour-led Government responded to the public outcry over National's half-cocked reforms by fudging and blurring the whole issue as much as they could. Helen Clark addressed the problem of waiting lists by refusing a place on the queue to anyone to whom the public system couldn't guarantee an operation within six months. Hey presto! You never heard of anyone waiting for more than six months for an operation any more! This was a master stroke by the mistress of political command and control. Amazingly, given the increasing numbers of people who had been tossed off the waiting lists for operations in the public system and who had no private health insurance, a charity hospital was once again established in Christchurch – the first in this country for 100 years (and another is planned for Auckland). History was repeating with a vengeance.

Labour also wound the clock back by returning to the local health board model (labelled District Health Boards, or DHBs this time round) and reversing the purchaser/provider split, charging locally elected boards with making local decisions on the prioritisation of resources. By having the 21 DHBs do the dirty work, central government politicians could keep their hands clean. The diffusion of responsibility across a plethora of parochial representatives was a return to the happy days before Kim Hill regularly pilloried the Minister of Health for public health sector failures on her Nine to Noon show on Radio New Zealand. The political sigh of relief from the Beehive was audible.

Mercifully for Labour, the economy was performing at long last, and awash with cash, the government could damp down the flames of discontent within the health system. It started spending on health, big time. Money and decentralisation obscured the whole prioritisation hot potato. The question of who got what care became fuzzier, but importantly, it became more and more difficult for the press to point the finger at anyone for denying necessary care. The newspapers fell meekly silent, save for the occasional bleat about waiting lists, and all the tough questions appeared to have gone away. The general public, who had only begun to face up to the cold realities of how thin the health budget was spread was able to return to its complacent sense of universal entitlement.

The only really strong prioritisation decision that the Labour-led Government made in healthcare was to place a new emphasis on primary care. The Primary Health Care Strategy was a bold attempt to reduce the cost of seeing your GP. Funding to GPs increased massively, but instead of paying per visit to your GP, each practice now got paid according to how many patients they have enrolled, regardless of how often the doctors are consulted. At the heart of this is the familiar notion that GPs should do well out of keeping you healthy, not just treating you. As we shall see in Chapter Four, there was a lot to be said for this policy from the perspectives of fairness and of catching health problems earlier. GPs were also encouraged to work together through Primary Health Organisations (PHOs), in order to improve services and coordination. PHOs work with GPs, nurses and other health professionals (such as physiotherapists and midwives) to plan and deliver healthcare services in the community to their enrolled patient base. As we'll see later, in a few areas PHOs have revolutionised the way primary care is delivered. In others, they just divvy up the cash amongst their member GPs.

So now, after three decades of revolution, the system looks pretty much the way it did in the late 1980s. The Minister of Health and his or her Ministry have overall responsibility for the 'health system'. The Ministry itself was largely spared from all the tortuous reforms inflicted on others during the Gibbs & Upton reform era. The hospitals in each of the 21 Health Districts are run by District Health Boards (DHBs), each with their own administration and Board (with a majority of members elected by the public). But DHBs aren't just the hospitals. DHBs are also responsible for preventing poor health among the people in their catchment area, and their funding is accordingly based on the size of their population base. To achieve their goals, the DHBs contract out or pass on money to others for some services – usually local stuff like GPs, midwives and diagnostic laboratories. GPs are still normally guys and gals running their own private business, unlike public hospitals, which remain publicly owned. Then, of course, there's the parallel universe of the private system, complete with its own privately owned hospitals, which are busy chipping away, doing their own thing. Operations in these hospitals are mostly funded by private medical insurance, although (as we've seen) ACC and the public system will occasionally buy their services, too.

If you think all this sounds confusing enough, remember that the 21 DHBs have 21 different ways of deciding how to spend, 21 different ways of collecting information and 21 different ways of running their hospitals. And all the private sector operators – GPs and private hospitals – do things their own way, too. GPs in particular don't always like to play ball with the latest government bright idea. After all, they have a business to run. No wonder there's variability in care around the country. It's really stretching the meaning of the words to say that we have one 'National Health System'. In fact, we have always had a loosely integrated multitude.

Summary

In sum, we have seen five stages in the evolution of our healthcare system, including a lot of action in the last twenty years:

i.   Pre 1938: Ad hoc Local Hospital Board System – managed by local authorities but various funding streams, including private and central government.

ii. 1938-1975: Nationalised System – Free hospital care funded by Department of Health through 30 Hospital Boards, with a subsidy for GP visits. Central funding disbursed through set formulae.

iii. 1975-1990: Gradual Shift to 14 Area Health Boards (AHB). This process began in 1975 but was not completed until 1988. Stronger accountability, population-based funding and focus on public health, not just running the hospital.

iv. 1990-1999: Regional Health Authority (RHA) and Crown Health Enterprise (CHE) model. Four RHAs purchased treatments off 23 CHEs and all GPs (to bargain collectively, GPs clubbed together in Independent Practitioner Associations – or IPAs). The four RHAs were briefly combined into a Health Funding Authority (HFA) at the end of the term.

v.   2000-present: The HFA was abolished. We moved to the District Health Board (DHB), of which there are 21, and Primary Health Organisation (of which there are over 80) model. This is largely a return to the AHB model, although there has been a significant change to GP payments, from a per-visit subsidy to funding based on enrolled patient base.

WHAT COST HEAL✚H?

There are three steps in assessing the quality of our health system. First, we'll look at how much we spend on health. Then we'll look at where it all goes. And then we'll need to try to measure the effectiveness of all this spending. This, as we'll see, is the hard part, because it's not just a simple matter of counting the number of hip operations, adding the number of paracetamol prescriptions and dividing by the annual health budget. Some quantitative analysis can be done; but most of what really counts is qualitative, and trying to generate hard data from studies of health and well-being is like trying to mount a jellyfish on a block of wood with a ramset gun.

Another Health Warning: Some of what you're about to read contains numbers, and the odd graph. But take a deep breath. It won't hurt a bit.

In looking at how the health system works, in terms of delivering health services to the population of New Zealand in return for cash, we'll be using a couple of terms that might need explanation up front.

To start with, we'll be talking about 'public health' from time to time. This is not to be confused with what we mean when we talk about the 'public health system'. Rather, it's what you might think of as the safety barrier at the top of the cliff of illness. It includes preventive measures, such as vaccination against infectious diseases, precautionary screening for others, education about keeping safe and healthy, and even such basic measures as sanitation.

As we talk it through, we'll be making a distinction between two aspects of providing health services: the funding (*purchasing*) on the one hand, and the real doctoring and nursing (*providing*) on the other. Private funding of healthcare may be done through private health insurance, where you pay a premium against the day you require medical treatment, whereupon your friendly insurance company happily pays for the treatment in full. That's the theory, anyway. But private funding can also be done on an ad hoc, 'out of pocket' basis, such as where you rock up to a GP and pay for a consultation, pay for a prescription at the chemist, or a blood test at the lab, or where you book yourself into a private clinic for a procedure, for example, without troubling the government or your medical insurer (assuming you have one). Public funding of healthcare is more familiar to us, because that's the way most of it is done in New Zealand. We pay taxes, and the government (more specifically, through the Ministry of Health) subsidises consultations with doctors, approved medications, and pays the hospital bills in full – pays for everything from the bricks and mortar, plant and equipment, the running and maintenance costs to the salaries of the medical and support staff.

When people talk about 'the health system', they generally mean all of the various components of however it is that New Zealanders set about getting health services delivered to them. As we've previously mentioned, New Zealand has a real mongrel of a health system, with a private component and an element of social insurance mixed in with the predominantly public system. And just to muddy the waters, there's some crossover: the 'social insurance' aspect (ACC) can purchase health services from both public and private providers. The public funding agencies (the Ministry of Health and DHBs) will sometimes purchase services from private providers, such as where they pay for operations in private hospitals.

Whew. OK. Clear on all that. So let's move on to look at how much New Zealanders spend on health, and how all that money gets to where it goes.

Totalling everything up, and according to the most recent figures available (2006), New Zealand spends around $15 billion on health every year, whether it be public money, or money disbursed by private insurance schemes or coughed up by patients out of their own pockets. The government finds most of this money ($12 billion) out of our taxes and ACC levies and disburses it through a number of agencies. The Ministry of Health handles around 65% of all money spent on health in New Zealand – 66% if you include the 1% that inevitably seems to be required to bail out indigent hospitals at the end of each financial year. The New Zealand public makes a cool $2.5 billion's worth of out-of-pocket expenditure, or 16% of the total. Private insurance accounts for just $724 million, or 5%, and charities contribute to a tiny, but not insignificant, degree too.

Figure 1   **Sources of healthcare funding (2005/06)**

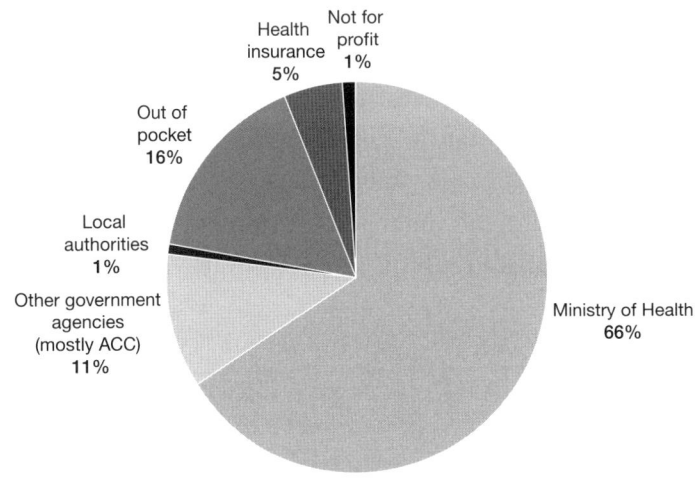

Source   Ministry of Health (2008)

The numbers have fluctuated in the last decade or so, naturally enough – the total health spend in 1984 was $2.2 billion – but so have the proportions, mainly due to the reforms of the intervening period. The government made significant cuts to its expenditure in the late 1980s and early 90s, and private insurance was the big winner, with around 45% of the population carrying some sort of private insurance at that time (at least, according to the industry). This trend slackened after 1996, and was dealt a major blow in the wake of our biggest private health insurer's Great Unilateral Variation of the Terms of Your Premium Contract Debacle of 2002 (see panel). For a time, Kiwis disposed to go private overwhelmingly preferred to pay out of pocket on an ad hoc, as-required basis rather than putting their trust in the promises of insurance companies again. Still, around a third of New Zealanders continue faithfully to fork out their monthly premium, although only 14% bother with comprehensive schemes (as opposed to cover against major events or treatments only). And if the industry is to be believed, the numbers are growing again, perhaps because there's a whole new generation of suckers, er, citizens whose memory doesn't stretch far enough back to be wary of how hollow 'whole-of-life' policy promises have proved.

So the first point to make about the funding of health services in New Zealand is that the government dominates it, through the disbursement of taxes and through ACC (which accounts for about 10% of total funding). Fully three quarters of all the money used to fund healthcare comes from the state.

Getting cross with Southern Cross

We have witnessed some of the problems with health insurance right here in New Zealand – as demonstrated by our own local favourite Southern Cross.

Southern Cross is a not-for-profit organisation that was established in 1979. With 14 hospitals and a shade over 800,000 members

(60% of the health insurance market) it is the largest provider of private insurance in the country.

Insurance works best when it includes lots of people who don't need it – so everyone is paying a little bit for their insurance cover. The original members of Southern Cross paid similar premiums regardless of age.

After a while, a system of three wide age bands was introduced. Premiums changed little under both approaches as premium-holders got older. Anyone with half a brain must have realised they were paying more than they needed to while they were young, in the expectation that they would pay less when they got older. In other words, there was an implicit cross-subsidy from younger members to older. This model must have appealed to those who wanted to smooth the cost of healthcare over a lifetime.

This business model proved to be unsustainable. By the 90s, the original baby boomer policyholders were growing older and were starting to use their insurance more to cover the inevitable hip and knee problems. Healthcare costs were also rising faster than originally predicted, and everyone's premiums had to rise in order to cover the cost. The cross-subsidy from young to old went up sixfold, and some premiums tripled as a result.

In 2002, the model of sharing risk across age-groups finally broke down completely. Young people were being scared off the scheme by the high premiums, and were going to other insurers offering lower rates or taking their chances with the public system. Southern Cross started charging different rates for every age, increasing charges for the elderly by up to 70% in a single year, all so they could offer a competitive rate for younger people. Price rises for older members have continued since then, including a 17% rise for customers over 70 in 2006.

Many elderly people – including those on lower incomes or in relatively good health – felt it wasn't worth paying the higher premiums. So they stopped paying, leaving behind the sicker premium payers, which inevitably meant costs kept rising... you get the picture. You can follow this process to the logical conclusion of insurance collapsing completely, with people paying premiums that are little short of the full user-pays rates for the services they consume. Insurance coverage dropped from about half of all New Zealanders in the early 90s to one third in the 2000s.

At least the way it worked out, Southern Cross kept its precious A+ financial rating from Standard and Poor's. Never mind about those pesky old folk.

Many original policyholders believe Southern Cross (and the insurance salesmen who sold them their policy) reneged on its promises, at least morally if not legally. If they'd been forced to honour their original premium structure, Southern Cross would almost certainly have gone under, creating huge disruption in the New Zealand insurance market. But maybe that way the public (and who knows, maybe even the management of Southern Cross) would have learned a hard lesson about the way private insurance works.

Health expenditure is growing at a rate that far outstrips our national income or our population growth. It's been growing at an average rate of 5% per annum since 1925. Indeed, over the last decade, the average increase in total health expenditure has been 6%, at a time when economic growth has barely managed half of that.

Put another way, our income per capita has increased at only 2.5% since 1995, and this is how it looks when we compare it graphically with what's been happening to our health expenditure:

Figure 2   **Growth in health spending outstrips income**

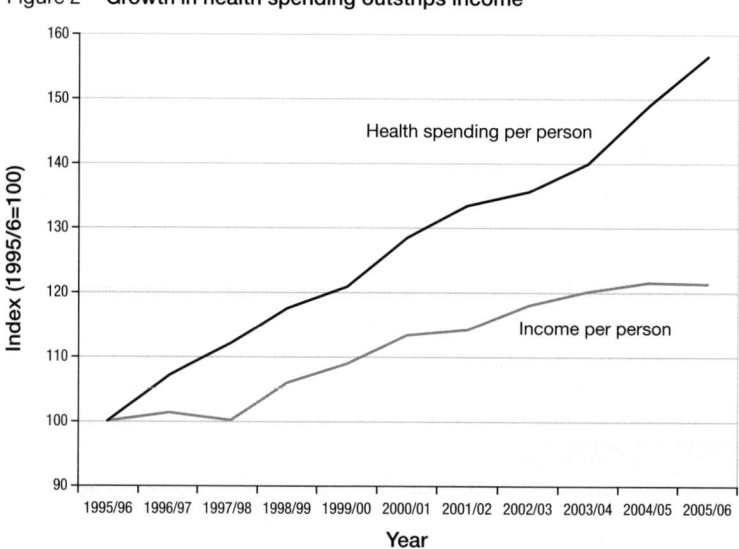

Source   Ministry of Health; Infometrics

Private spending has increased, but not that fast. So the shortfall has necessarily been made up out of the public purse. The government has been forced to spend more and more on health every year. That makes for another scary graph:

Figure 3 **Health spending growth since 1925**

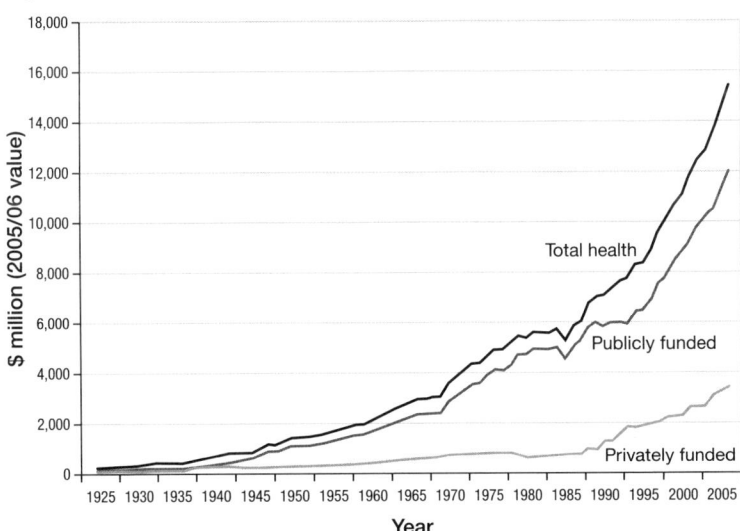

Source   Ministry of Health (2008)

So the second point to make is that the government's commitment to doing the lion's share of healthcare funding has cost it more and more dearly as the years have gone by. Nor is the prognosis very good. It's projected that at the current rate of increase, the percentage of national income gobbled up by health expenditure will double to 12% by 2050.

Keeping Up with the Joneses
How does the amount we spend on healthcare stack up internationally – or at least (since there's little reason comparing our health system with, say, Gabon's), by comparison with the

rest of the developed world?

New Zealanders spent the equivalent of US$2,211 per capita in 2006. That placed us 20th in the list of big spenders, way behind the United States (US$6000 per capita) and behind most of the European nations, but roughly comparable to Australia and the United Kingdom. In terms of what proportion of our national income (or Gross Domestic Product) we spent, the picture was broadly similar: we were bang on the 2006 OECD average for health expenditure as a percentage of GDP, namely 9.6%. To put it in perspective, America spends fully 15% – one dollar in every seven earned – on healthcare, whereas the European nations average out at roughly 11% amongst themselves.

So we can hardly be accused of being extravagant, even if the proportion of our national income spent on healthcare has been growing more quickly than the OECD average since 1995 (which merely signifies that we've been catching up since the government came over all stingy in the 'reform era', 1987-1994). The rough uniformity of the numbers suggests that there's some kind of 'natural' limit to the amount a developed nation spends on health, and if this is so, then the key to meeting increased costs in the healthcare sector must lie in boosting national income.

This lesson is especially true for New Zealand. While we spend the bog-standard, general-issue, OECD-average proportion of our national income on health, we have to remember at all times that we just don't earn that much. If you've decided you're going to spend 10% of your annual salary on a new car and you earn $70,000 a year, you're not going to be driving anything quite as snazzy as the bloke on $700,000 per annum who makes the same proportional commitment. It's the same in healthcare, because we're shopping in a global market. 9.6% of New Zealand's GDP of US$115 billion isn't going to get us a Rolls Royce healthcare system when we're competing with, say, Australia, with a GDP of US$795 billion.

Slicing it up

Where does all that money go? How is it apportioned?

The short answer is that most of it ($7.4 billion in 2006) goes on *primary care*, by which is meant visits to doctors, paying for prescriptions from pharmacies, diagnostic tests and other services, such as home-based healthcare, physiotherapists, outpatient services, dentists and so on. Of this, 37% of the tab was picked up by the private sector, and the lion's share of this will have been through patients digging into their own pockets to pay their GP, their pharmacist and the diagnostic laboratory. Primary care is subsidised in New Zealand: your doctor didn't get his Porsche and his six-monthly overseas golfing holidays simply by putting every $30 consultation fee in a jar somewhere. The government picks up the rest of his bill, as it has done ever since Michael Joseph Savage first decided they should in 1938. Similarly, the cost of the drugs you get on prescription is heavily subsidised – provided, of course, they're in Pharmac's good books.

The next biggest recipient is the combination of *secondary* and *tertiary care*, by which is meant intensive treatment after diagnosis (usually in a hospital, and often involving highly specialised equipment and personnel). Of the $5.1 billion spent in this area in 2006, 12% was forked out by the private sector. This almost certainly represents the purchase of operations in private hospitals and clinics by private insurers.

Next biggest is nursing and residential care, such as where a District Nurse visits the elderly and the infirm being cared for in their own homes. There are private agencies that do this kind of work, but in New Zealand, their combined activity accounts for only 1% of the $1.5 billion spent annually. The state funds most of the rest. Public health and the administration of the health system account for roughly 6% and 4% of total expenditure respectively.

Figure 4   **Where the money goes**

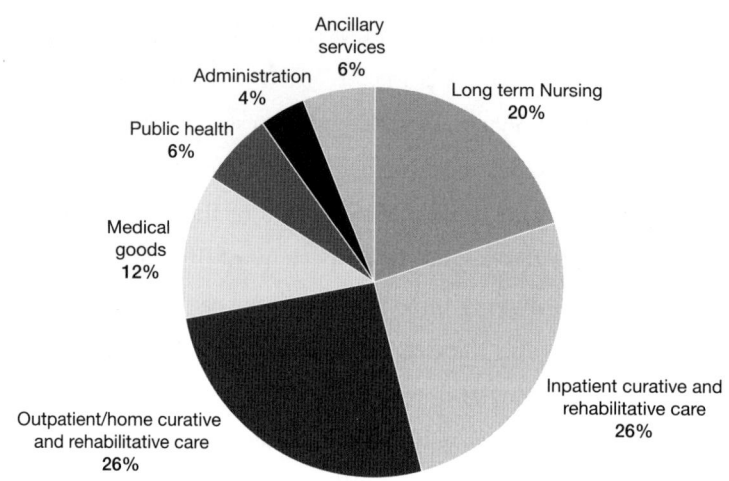

Source   Ministry of Health (2008)

New Zealand is notable in spending more on public health and prevention than other countries, and less on dental care. Savage had intended dental care to be included in his fully-funded public health system, but he was voted down. Consequently, in New Zealand, dental care for anyone over 18 has traditionally been delivered by the private sector and funded directly out of people's pockets. The relatively high level of funding for public health ought to be a good thing, given how convinced the health professionals we spoke to were that expenditure in this area would return the greatest bang for the health buck. It really is more rewarding to put a barrier at the top of the cliff, that is, than just to pay for ambulances to queue up at the bottom.

New Zealand is also somewhat unusual in that it has managed to slow down the growth of pharmaceutical spending over recent years. It actually makes up a lower proportion of total health spending than it did in 1996 – just over 12%, down from almost 15% in 1996.[12] Meanwhile, the pharmaceutical budgets of our competitors are soaring: the OECD average spending on drugs rose from 14% to 16.4%. This is largely due to the success of Pharmac. Pity, then, that John Key's first contribution to the health sector was to undermine Pharmac.

Finding and keeping quality staff is a challenge in any industry, but in the health sector, the challenges are even greater. New Zealand is competing with a large – and richer – English-speaking market for health staff. It seems there are staff shortages everywhere you look – Britain, US, Australia and Canada.

Is there a doctor in the house?

We're far below the OECD average for doctor numbers, but relatively flush for nurses. This data comes with an important proviso. In part, the difference reflects the European obsession with employing doctors, whereas Anglo countries tend to employ fewer doctors and instead to employ more nurses. All the same, we have slightly fewer doctors than other Anglo countries, and while doctor and nurse numbers have been steadily growing, the rate has also been below the OECD average.

Our GP base is similar to that in the rest of the OECD, but comparatively speaking, we have significantly fewer specialists. This is probably what accounts for the six-month period you're frequently obliged to wait simply to see a specialist – never mind the wait involved once he or she has put you on the list for elective surgery. Sheesh! We're waiting to wait!

The importance of incentives – where did all the GPs go?

While absolute numbers of GPs are comparable with elsewhere in the world, the spread of practices is not even across the country. In the past, this has created some access problems.

Part of the rationale for the fifth Labour-led government's primary healthcare reforms was to address the dearth of GPs in poor areas.

The reason for this is that the majority of GP income previously came from charges to their customers. Why would a GP set up in a poor area when they will have a much better income from less work as a result of operating in a wealthy area? The financial incentive to avoid the slums has been effective. The DHBs with the fewest GPs per head of population are Taranaki, West Coast and Counties Manukau – all relatively poor or remote areas. But on a district council basis, it is the poor and rural Opotiki that has the fewest GPs per head of population with less than ¼ of the national average.[13]

Helen Clark's government tried to deal with this by paying GPs on the basis of their enrolled population, rather than per visit. Funding was adjusted for higher risk groups, to encourage GPs to operate in these areas.

All the same, the General Practice side of the health system is on the brink of another and far worse crisis. Everyone knows our population is ageing, but we seldom stop to consider how many doctors are due to retire precisely as the rest of the population is going to start banging on their door.

The old chestnut raised by the medical unions is pay. They claim that if we pay doctors and nurses competitive rates, then they will stick around. Interestingly, when you compare their salaries to other New Zealanders, doctors and nurses here get paid pretty well – for example, pay packets for nurses are above the OECD average as a share of national income.[14] But we simply can't compete with the pay packets in the US, UK and Australia. The trouble again is that our national income is lower than that of our English-speaking competitors, so other places can afford to pay their doctors more. Just as we can attract Filipino nurses with our standard of living, so our doctors and nurses are often enticed by the bright lights of London, New York and (for some reason) Sydney. A recent Commission found that senior doctors were getting offered 30-35% higher pay to ply their trade across the Tasman.[15] The majority of this difference in pay packets can be explained by the difference in Australia's average income per capita – it's just higher than ours. So we're like a poker player with their last chip – if we try to raise the pay stakes we'll get out-bid.

This quandary can be seen more clearly in the context of recent health sector spending increases. Under the Labour-led Government, health spending grew faster than it had ever done before. However, around 60% of the recent spending increase has gone on personnel, and the majority of this has gone into paying existing staff more rather than recruiting more staff. Our hospitals are in a cleft stick here. To attract staff from overseas, they will need to pay more. If they pay more, they're faced with the need to pay everyone more. We'll look at the issue of finding and keeping medical staff in more detail in Chapter 7.

Bricks and mortar

Let's turn now to the facilities from which our medical services are delivered. It's pretty difficult to compare the quality of hospitals internationally, unless you're as accident-prone as you're widely travelled. The only measure that can be used as a basis for comparison is the number of hospital beds. According to the World Health Organisation,[16] we have more hospital beds per capita than other Anglo countries, but fewer than the likes of Japan. Quite obviously, this is our first brush with the problem of qualitative versus quantitative measures: it's not always true to say that more beds mean better healthcare. But neither is it true to say a flash new hospital provides better healthcare than a tired, dilapidated one: what matters is the services provided. An expert we spoke to talked of Oxford Hospital, parts of which have been standing in need of TLC since World War II – peeling paint, broken fittings, buckets to catch drips in the corridors – but where the services offered were outstanding, making it an exhilarating place for staff to work. Another told us that in her area, there are too few staff to provide services in the grand facilities that had just been built. There's more to making a new hospital work than simply cutting a ribbon.

Machines that go 'Ka-ching!'

Finally, we're below the OECD average in the use of the new-fangled tools of the trade such as CT scanners, and well below in terms of MRI units. The mammography and radiation therapy units, on the other hand, are above average.[17] Lack of technology isn't always a bad thing: doctors have their boys' toys, too, and some have a fetish for the latest gadgets regardless of their return on investment. Our relative lack of machines may also be nothing more than a simple reflection of our lack of scale. After all, New Zealand's health system serves a population little bigger than that of a medium-sized city overseas, and some specialised machines would never see enough use to justify the expense. Of more concern is the way in which the machines we do have are acquired and used. The DHBs don't play well together, and prefer each to buy their own little toys to play with rather than pitching in for one really good sandpit they can all use. As a result, fragmentation and the lack of coordination may cost us the opportunity to acquire major diagnostic machines that could, in turn, benefit New Zealand as a whole.

National service and technology review committee

New Zealand is lucky enough to have a Committee with a moniker to rival NASA – the National Service and Technology Review (NSTR) Committee. This is a group that prioritises new health technology at a national level. Some of the brightest minds in the medical profession examine the evidence and make recommendations about what new healthcare technology we should take up.

Sounds great, right? They come up with some pretty good recommendations. The only problem is they have no real power. Their recommendations are met with earnest nods from the Ministry of Health, and glazed eyes from the DHBs (who actually control the money).

Take PET/CT scanning (positron emission tomography and computed axial tomograph, if you must know). This uses fluorodeoxyglucose (FDG) – radioactive glucose – to provide immensely high-resolution 'maps' of a patient's metabolism, including abnormalities such as cancerous cells, within the body, allowing tumours to be precisely cut out or zapped without taking out great tracts of sound tissue as collateral damage. Previously patients were sent to Australia for this diagnostic service. NSTR recommended establishing three scanners in NZ, with an additional unit in Auckland to provide the FDG needed to run the scanners. However, despite convincing evidence of clinical benefit and cost-effectiveness for New Zealand patients, the DHBs couldn't agree to pitch in for a new service that would end up being based in Auckland. Eventually, a private operator brought in a scanner and the DHBs now purchase the service off an outfit that's based in Wellington – for a small fee, of course…

So the last point to make in relation to the inputs into the New Zealand health system – the fiscal and the physical – is this. In *relative* spending terms, we spend exactly the proportion of our income that you would expect, and on roughly the range of things that you would expect. But in *absolute* terms, we spend less on healthcare than other OECD nations. Compared to other rich countries, such as our trans-Tasman rival, New Zealand runs its health system on the smell of an oily rag. The simple truth is that we can't afford to spend much more than we do because we're a poorer nation. If we want First World healthcare, then first and foremost, we have to make sure we maintain a First World income.

What do we get for our money?

Now that we've seen what goes into the health system, let's see what we get out of it. There are two stages to this process. The first stage is to look at the system's outputs, the crude, quantitative measures of health sector productivity that are available. The remainder of this chapter will be devoted to this discussion.

The second stage is to look at the best available indicators of the system's effectiveness, and for a health system, that surely has to be how healthy we are as a nation. That's what we'll proceed to do in the next chapter.

Outputs can be difficult to compare. Simply counting the numbers of operations your money buys doesn't tell you much. If your hip replacement budget seems to have bought you surprisingly few procedures, it doesn't necessarily mean you've been sold a pup. On the contrary, the operations that were performed may have been more difficult and yet more valuable, perhaps because (say) they got younger people back into a state of productive health. And getting loads and loads of operations for your outlay may even be a bad thing, as when, say, the procedures were unnecessary. What's more, the better your preventive measures, the fewer medical interventions will be required, but while your health system will be doing the best possible job, the operation-counting approach will find it wanting.

The data can be ambiguous. New Zealanders have dramatically fewer consultations (just under four a year) with doctors than most other OECD nations (most Europeans and your average Australian see their doctor six times a year; Japanese say 'Aaaah' – in Japanese, of course – 14 times a year). So what does the number mean? We have so few doctors that we can only track one down four times a year? We're willing to let practice nurses handle much of the stuff that everyone else in the developed world has to see a doctor about? One would be a bad thing. The other would be good. So which is it?

Even where you can devise a meaningful performance criterion for your health system, international comparison data is difficult to collect. In some cases, it is less than reliable. In others, it takes many years to put together and can be out of date by the time it is published. This leaves you with no way of knowing whether your own system's performance is acceptable in the international context, or whether you're living in a fool's paradise.

Another major problem with output data, and particularly the output data that is used to frame international comparisons, is that it focuses heavily on what happens in hospitals. As we've seen above, our health system is much more than this. The safety barrier at the top, the public health measures and the primary system, are at least as important – you'll find plenty of experts who argue they're far *more* important – than what happens at the bottom of the cliff.

Out, Patients!

Still, the international comparisons of hospital-based data will reveal any major anomalies in a resource-intensive area of the sector. The comparisons are worth a look.

One way to judge how busy your hospitals are is to count the number of patients they discharge. You're presuming they're not burying or burning a large proportion of those they're admitting, but it's to be expected that you're also counting those!

The international data on hospital discharges suggests that New Zealand is just below the OECD average in terms of discharges, although not far behind the pack. If you compare this to the *absolute* amount we spend on healthcare, New Zealand seems efficient. The average cost per discharge is around US$4900 compared to the OECD median of US$6400.[18] However, in *relative* terms, we spend the average amount of our national income and deliver a below-average number of operations. This suggests the cost of operations in New Zealand is out of line with the average costs of this economy. Operations are relatively expensive on the international scale.

But let's not push the data too hard. Not all hospital discharges are the same. We may do more complex procedures compared to overseas averages. This might explain the disparity, but to know for sure, we'd need finer data, and it just doesn't exist. We can, to a limited extent, make like-for-like comparisons across individual procedures, as each procedure should cost the same on average. But no sooner do you embark, fresh-faced and bushy-tailed, on this kind of endeavour than the caveats come crowding in. No two procedures are the same: some are more complex than others, for reasons that are inscrutable to the data collector.

Anyway, leaving aside all that fuzziness, for most procedures where there is data, New Zealand performs fewer per capita than the OECD average. Don't panic: this could mean something good. It could mean that our larger spend on public health makes a lot of hospital care unnecessary – fewer bodies at the bottom of the cliff. It could mean something more neutral: we have a higher threshold for deeming surgical intervention necessary.

Then again, of course, it could mean something bad, such as that we can't afford as many operations as we'd like to fund because of our lower national income means lower investment in healthcare.

Let's put some numbers to all this. We in New Zealand tend to do only half as much cancer treatment as the OECD average. We do about a third less treatment of heart disease and strokes. As we'll see, diabetes and mental health problems are growing rapidly, but we do only three quarters as much for sufferers of these conditions as the average OECD country. We're going to go on and look at what ails (and kills us) in the next chapter, but suffice to say here that our rates of diabetes, mental illness, and our death rates from cancer and heart disease, are all above the OECD average, so it seems unlikely our lower rate of procedures is due to a lower need for treatment. Indeed, New Zealand doctors have to deal with higher rates of emergency heart attacks – 50% more than other countries. It looks very much as though the only factor that can explain our lower procedure rates is funding. New Zealand is too poor to afford all the treatments we might want. Compared to richer countries, we have unmet health needs.

A quick tip for all those future doctors and nurses out there, wondering where they should specialise. The data is pretty limited, but everything indicates that obesity and ageing will be the drivers of future diseases. Diabetes and Alzheimer's disease are the fastest expanding areas. We've seen big falls in numbers treated for cataracts and angina. In the case of cataract operations, at least, there's no reason to believe that this signifies a fall in demand. It's more likely to be down to the scarcity of resources – although pricing by the cartel of ophthalmologists may have something to do with it, too. Still, either way, not a great result for those losing their sight to this easily treatable condition.[19]

One problem with our low treatment rates is that it becomes common for single-issue groups to attract media attention to our poor performance relative to Australia in respect of this or that procedure. Over the past year alone, reports have been released fulminating on our lower rates of treatment for heart disease and respiratory problems. It may well make sense to increase one or more of these treatments, depending on the relative improvement in health for a given cost. Certainly, if you're a politician in search of an instant boost in popularity, it will make perfect sense to divert a few resources to the problem area. But this, above all, is where the big picture approach is needed. We're a poorer nation than Australia, and than most of the nations to whom we compare ourselves in the OECD, for that matter. Without higher economic growth, it will simply be impossible to match them. The squeaky wheel approach to funding – and it's proved irresistible to a succession of Ministers – is doomed to cast our Health Minister as a clown prodding a balloon, pressing down on one issue only to see the system ballooning out elsewhere. A 'big push' in one area is invariably at the expense of other parts of the health system, which inevitably end up on the front page in two years' time. And so the wheel turns.

There's definitely some good news buried amongst all the doom and gloom of this international comparative stuff. As mentioned, New Zealand spends more on prevention than most countries, and this fact is borne out by the number of preventative treatments undertaken. We do pretty well when it comes to jabbing older people for the flu in wintertime. Likewise, our screening programmes for diseases like breast cancer and cervical cancer are clearly world class, as we're above international averages for the take-up. The only glaring exception to our excellent public health performance is childhood vaccinations. We are among the lowest in the OECD for sticking needles in our kids. Does this reflect popular cynicism and mistrust of vaccination? After all, for every new vaccine made available, there always seems to be a high-profile scare campaign linking it to all manner of ghastly potential side-effects – just look at the hue and cry raised over the (spurious) link between the MMR (measles, mumps, rubella) jab for infants and autism. Vaccination rates are lowest amongst poorer communities – 71% of kids under two are immunised in poor areas and the rates are even lower for Maori (68%), compared to 82% in rich areas.[20] This suggests that the young and poor are missing out as the old, grumpy and privileged are capturing the resources, rather than a mistrust of vaccination more generally. As we'll see, that the poor, young and voiceless (especially Maori) are missing out to the clamouring, middle-class, blue-rinsed masses is a common theme in the health sector.

Taking to our beds

What else can we find out about how effectively our health dollar is being spent?

We've already looked at the number of hospital beds, and

we've seen that we compare pretty well in terms of the number of beds we get for our buck. But as with most of these measures, this is ambiguous. A hospital bed can only fit one person at a time, so your ability to treat new patients is limited by your ability to discharge old patients. If you're turning people over really fast, you can treat more people. But as you can readily see, this isn't necessarily a great indicator of the quality of care. If all your patients are being discharged straight into the cemetery, for example, or if they're back after a week because post-operative complications have set in, you can hardly be said to be running an effective health system, no matter how good it looks on this particular bit of paper. We've all heard horror stories of friends turfed out of a hospital seconds after an operation or just after having given birth. At times, it seems new mothers are sent home faster than you can say 'postnatal depression'. No one disputes that hospital beds are a precious resource, but it offends our sensibilities to be treated as though we're cows at the milking shed.

Nonetheless, average length of stay is another internationally recognised measure of hospital efficiency. The shorter a person's stay in a hospital bed, the more treatments can happen. Again, comparisons are difficult because treatments may be different, but New Zealand's Average Length of Stay (ALOS) for inpatients (those who stay overnight) indicates that we have a shorter length of stay (just over seven days) than most other nations. Australians loll about for a fortnight on average, and the Japanese for over a month. It may have something to do with the food.

And our ALOS for all patients (a slightly different measure to the international comparisons above) has been steadily falling over time – from just over seven days in 1988 to just over four days more recently. However, there is high variability across hospitals on this measure. Comparisons are difficult, as simpler procedures require less bed rest and monitoring than complex ones. Without knowing in detail what kind of procedures are being tackled, it's hard to be definitive about this measure. Still, the range is suspicious. The longest ALOS is 30% higher than the smallest ALOS.[21] There seems to be obvious potential to increase the numbers of treatments in certain hospitals. Let's not beat around the bush. Here are the names of our 'Hospital Hiltons': Capital and Coast, Waikato, Otago and Mid-Central DHBs have some explaining to do.

If the ghastly anecdotal evidence is true, and we really do wheel people out into the street and tip them off the gurney before they're fully out from under the general anaesthetic, then we've been really lucky with the outcomes. Our relatively short ALOS generally doesn't seem to compromise the quality of our healthcare.[22] Survival rates after treatment are generally good compared to other countries. This is one of the best places in the world to suffer a heart attack or be admitted for surgery on colorectal cancer – we're above average in these areas, probably (and tragically) because our doctors get so much practice in them. On the other hand, we don't look so good when it comes to dealing with strokes and asthma.

Whoops!

A related issue is the so-called *iatrogenic artefact*, the fancy term medical men and women like to use to refer to medical cock-ups. New Zealand research indicates that around 13% of hospital admissions are due to problems arising from medical treatment. 'Surgical precision' is sometimes a contradiction in terms. Just under 15% of these incidents were serious, resulting in some permanent disability or death. This means that just under 2% of people receiving medical treatment are likely to suffer serious harm from that 'care'.[23] But as high as this figure seems, it's pretty much in line with overseas results. Hospitals are busy places, with a lot going on, and a lot can go wrong, not least the contracting of hospital-based infections. We will look at this issue again in Chapter Eight.

Wake up, Doc

Data collection to measure the productivity of health professionals is pretty recent and is something of a blunt instrument. It links spending with outputs (such as the number of operations, for example) rather than with outcomes (such as people living longer, healthier or fuller lives), which would seem far more important. There's no adjustment for other qualitative measures, such as patient satisfaction, or even mortality. And the data is patchy at best: it only covers some aspects of inpatient surgery (it omits outpatient work completely), and the quality of data can vary widely across hospitals.

But based on these data, Treasury, Ministry of Health and Business Roundtable estimates all suggest that the cost per procedure in this country has gone up since 2000, resulting in fewer procedures performed per buck spent on hospitals. Most of this cost has been absorbed by the wage and salary bill, which has grown by around 40% since 2001/02. Outputs, meanwhile, only grew by about 10%. This means that the cost per output (i.e. procedure) has grown by about 30%. Some studies indicate that this result is also consistent with the experience of the 1990s.[24] Overall, this suggests that to increase hospital outputs in New Zealand by 1% requires a whopping funding increase of 3%. This may be partly due to inefficiencies, but also seems due to the tight market for medical staff. To do more operations we need more staff. To attract more staff we need to increase wages.

We shouldn't beat ourselves up about it too much. Exactly the same pattern has been observed in the UK. Difficulties in increasing staff numbers saw health output (operations etc) per worker plummet by 8% between 2001 and 2006. Despite funding increases of almost 30% over these years, National Health Service

(NHS) output rose less than 20%. As in New Zealand, the reason seems to be that the NHS was spending too much of its increased budget trying to retain existing staff let alone to recruit the new staff it needed to do more operations.[25] It seems international competition for health professionals is being felt and we get less per dollar spent in this area now.

More worrying, productivity per staff member seems to have fallen over the period in which it has been measured.[26] Each staff member is achieving less with his or her day at the mill. There could be many reasons for this. It may reflect the additional 'non-work' demands that staff unions have extracted from DHBs over the period, which may reduce the amount of time spent doing 'productive' work. The hordes of new doctors and nurses employed may be less productive than the ones already preceding them in the system. Maybe the modern doctor or nurse spends more of their day filling out forms, or doing stuff not regarded by flinty-hearted Treasury officials as 'productive', such as sitting and holding patients' hands. The final (and most likely explanation) is that all the cash poured in by Labour over the noughties (i.e. 2000-2008) took the pressure off hospitals to be efficient. As a result a proportion of the money injected by Labour has probably been wasted.

It's also possible that data problems mean the results have failed to detect some part of the return on the investment, such as increased outpatient activity, or an improvement in quality of the outputs. Nevertheless, the initial signs are not encouraging, given all the money allocated. The Labour-led Government increased spending by $5 billion between 1999 and 2008 – roughly doubling the total health spend – and this over a period in which our income increased by only 60%. Surely New Zealanders have a right to know what they're getting in exchange for all the hard-earned tax dollars that have been pumped into the veins of the health system over the last few years.

Summary

In this chapter, we've looked at how we arrange to fund our health services, and what we get for the money we spend. Overwhelmingly, we fund the health system through the state, although we carry a small amount of private insurance and, when need arises, we dig into our pockets to pay directly. We spend neither more nor less of our national income than most of the rest of the developed world on healthcare, but of course, our income is lower than most. This accounts for the fact that we do fewer procedures in New Zealand than they do in comparable developed nations. Still, although the overall number of procedures we perform is below average, the quality of our procedures is not.

The most worrying element of New Zealand's hospital performance is how little outputs have increased in recent years despite the additional funding put into the sector. This recent injection of funding gives us some idea of how much we get back from putting new money into healthcare. The answer is 'a bit, but not much'.

Knowing about the quality of New Zealand care is useful. We already know that our system is relatively efficient – we produce a good number of hospital procedures for the money put in. If we know that these procedures are generally of an international standard then we can be assured this efficiency doesn't come at the price of cutting too many corners.

Economists always get hassled about knowing the cost of everything and the value of nothing. So let's give the health sector some credit. It creates enormous value. It keeps us alive longer for starters, which is pretty cool. But longer life gives us more than another year or two of playing golf. Healthcare really is an investment – not only is it a source of innovation in its own right, but when people live longer they invest more in things like their education and their retirement savings. This makes us all richer.[27] So the most meaningful measurement of the effectiveness of the health system can only be the health of the nation.

Come on, New Zealand. Slip off your shirt and climb up on the table. It's time for your physical.

The placebo effect

Emma is three years old, with a shock of curly brown hair, sun-kissed cheeks and a bewitching smile. She can't say the letter S yet, but she is grown up enough to play outside with her big sister. The risk of doing big sister things though is that she can very easily hurt herself. And she often does. When this happens, Emma then runs inside (with a speed belying the apparent injury), curls up on Mummy's lap and the floods of tears begin. There is no blood, but the anguish on Emma's face appears to indicate a broken bone at the very least.

In the past a cuddle and a magic kiss to the affected area would suffice. But Emma is past believing in magic kisses. Now she believes in the miracles of modern medicine. She will not stop crying until a band aid is applied to the affected area. Once applied, her tears abate, and she takes a moment to admire the wonder cure, which she will later show off to her sister as a battle scar.

The question is, do we really grow out of this childlike naïvety when it comes to medicine? We like to think of our doctors as infallible, and rigidly believe that if we follow their instructions to the letter we will be cured. Alas, sometimes we are mistaken, but most of the time we are not. The question is whether this is testimony to the skill of our doctors or the placebo effect.

The placebo effect occurs when the *results of a treatment come from a means other than its direct physiological reaction'.*[28] One of the great mysteries of modern medicine is the incredible ability of the mind to heal the body when given an excuse to do so. Simply by people believing they will be cured can create such a reaction. The triggers are hardly more sophisticated than Emma's sticking plaster – a brightly coloured sugar pill, sham surgery (giving someone a scar and telling them they have been operated on) or even a prayer all seem to do the trick. Provided, of course, that the patient (and ideally the doctor) believes in the cure.

The placebo effect is possibly the most powerful force in all medicine – both modern and ancient. Simply because it is isolated by modern science doesn't mean it doesn't still hold a powerful sway over the medical industry.

Studies of the potency of the placebo effect show it can account for *between one third and two thirds* of the successful treatment outcomes.[29] Astounding.

The placebo effect can work both ways. As strokes became preventable in the 1960s the debate raged about what was considered 'high' blood pressure, and therefore who should be treated with the new drugs that were available. Much to the delight of the pharmaceutical industry, high blood pressure was defined to be 'above average' blood pressure, thereby instantly diagnosing just under half the population with an with an arbitrary and, by definition, artificial illness. This had huge cost in dispensing drug treatments, but also impacted on people's health. Having been diagnosed with high blood pressure, steel workers in the US had dramatically higher rates of absenteeism – purely because they had been labelled as 'ill'.[30]

It is indeed a quirky consequence of how we measure health sector inputs, outputs and outcomes that the placebo effect may be the single most powerful healer of people, but it is deemed worthless because the impact is only in the patient's mind. Scientific tests are designed to isolate and exclude the placebo effect, yet we don't really know how it works. Despite their effectiveness, using placebos opens up all sorts of ethical problems for the modern professional doctor. After all, for the placebo to work, the doctor has to correctly identify the patient's 'illness' as being psychosomatic. You wonder how many GPs are trained to identify that.

The placebo effect may explain the occasional success of alternative 'fringe' treatments. Not bounded by scientific rigour or the Hippocratic Oath, alternative practitioners can more easily work with a person's belief system, as did the faith healers of old. It makes you wonder why our health system avoids making use of the healing powers of mind over matter when they could well be stronger than modern medicine. Perhaps there is nothing wrong with occasionally harnessing the placebo effect. Just ask Emma.

Chapter 3

YOUR HEAL✝H, NEW ZEALAND

In the end, the health of the population is the best measure of the effectiveness of health spending. It's a more holistic measure than the dry (and ambiguous) statistics we were examining in the previous chapter, and it has the advantage of capturing the effect of the public health measures we pay for as well. For while most of the media coverage around 'the health system' tends to focus on hospitals, there's more to keeping us alive and healthy than how many punters you're slicing and dicing.

But how do you measure how healthy we are? Assessing the *outcomes* of health spending is just as fraught as measuring *outputs*. There are some quantitative measurements available. One of the most basic measures used to determine the health of a nation is Average Life Expectancy at Birth. As the name suggests, that's how long you can expect to live, statistically speaking, if you survive the birth process. It's not underwritten by any kind of government guarantee, of course, and the rosy glow of a good number can actually conceal some nasty disorders, as we'll show when we come to consider Maori health. But broadly speaking, if your population's life expectancy is going up, your efforts to improve the health and well-being of your people are likely to be paying off. And since life expectancy can be compared across borders, it can also give you some idea of how efficient your healthcare system is relative to other countries.

We'll have a look at the life expectancy of New Zealanders in this chapter – what has been the trend in the average span of our lives relative to other countries, and relative to what we spend on health. We'll also have a look behind the capital number, at life expectancies by gender, ethnicity and income, because if we can work an improvement in any given group in society, our overall number will reflect it. The converse is also true. If any given group in society is dropping dead sooner than they should – letting the side down – they're making us look bad on the world stage.

Besides the crude indicator that is life expectancy, there's a survey of countries that has been ranking their health systems according to a number of criteria since 2004. The bad news is that the survey only takes in six countries; the good news is that New Zealand is one of these. It will be useful to have a peek at how we're doing by this reckoning, too.

And along the way, we'll have a look at some of the things that are within our control and that can jeopardise our health – our 'risk indicators', or unhealthy practices – and also go through the leading killers of Kiwis.

By the time we've finished looking at the health of the nation, we'll have arrived at some understanding of how much benefit we receive from the heavy cost that we incur to fund our health system. We'll have a pretty good handle on what kind of shape it's in, that is, and this will stand us in good stead when we move on to look at what challenges it's going to face in the near future.

How long, O Lord?

Way back in 1899, when the first contingent of New Zealanders and Australians disembarked from their troop transports in Cape Town, the British officers who saw them were stunned. These tall, buff, bronzed gods of men were a far cry from the weedy, hollow-chested specimens under their own command, whose Imperial Red uniforms didn't exactly show their pasty complexions to their best advantage. All-in-all, the physical shape the colonials were in was a wonderful advertisement for the health benefits of emigration.

The same impression was made when the 1905 All Blacks – the 'Originals' – toured the British Isles, trampling the pride of English manhood underfoot on their way to a record of 31 wins and but a single loss – and that the result of a combination of Welsh skulduggery and the incompetence of a Scottish referee. The English papers of the day were full of anguished reflection on why it was that the once-mighty English race had degenerated, whereas the rude colonials had gone ahead so. The New Zealand Prime Minister, Richard 'King Dick' Seddon, meanwhile, was happily taking out advertisements in the same newspapers proclaiming New Zealand's natural advantages, and the salutary effect of the Kiwi way of life. New Zealand was god's own country.

And all that, remember, was before we had a health system worthy of the name.

Only fifty years before, life expectancy was just 40 years, much as it had been in Europe from the Middle Ages right through to Victorian times. That's a pretty low number. It suggests that a high proportion of our ancestors celebrated their 21st and their parents' funerals within a fairly short space of time! But of course, it's an average. It reflects the dismal numbers of people who died in their infancy or early childhood, and obscures the fact that many New Zealanders – about a third – managed to live comfortably into their sixties or even higher. And herein lies the first clue about life expectancy numbers. Change something significant in part of the population – reduce the rate of infant mortality, for example – and you can do wonders for your rankings in the international life expectancy stakes.

For each decade that has passed since 1850, life expectancy has risen by two years. That's like getting a bonus weekend tacked onto your life every two working weeks! But the greater part of the dramatic increase in life expectancy that occurred between 1850 and (roughly) 1950 had to do with public health rather than with healthcare in the narrow sense. Improvements in housing, the hygiene and quality of food and water, sanitation and effective measures for the control of infectious diseases all contributed, especially to a drop in infant mortality. In fact, it's reckoned that of the 30-year surge in life expectancies that occurred in the hundred years between 1850 and 1950, only five can actually be attributed to healthcare.

But in the early years of the twentieth century, it was found that simply shovelling more money into this area didn't produce anything like the same returns. By the early years of the twentieth century, that is, the major advances in public health had all been made. Here was a classic case of what economists call 'diminishing marginal returns': increased investment yields ever greater results, but only up to a point. Beyond that point, each unit more in investment yields progressively less return.

After World War II, the rise of medicine began to make more of an impact, reducing mortality from a range of illnesses and injuries. The rise of modern medicine has been portrayed as the triumph of science over pesky microscopic critters. This created the impression that by shovelling more dosh at men in white coats, we could smash a wider range of critters and live forever. In reality most 'breakthroughs' were either flukes or the result of exhaustive trial and error: penicillin was discovered in dirty petri dishes left over the summer holidays (and it took ten years for anyone to realise it might be useful), while chemotherapy started off as a side-effect of exposure to mustard gas and had to be painstakingly refined until it didn't kill quite so many people. Incredibly, modern medicine still doesn't really understand the causes of most of our major ailments, nor why a lot of the treatments we have discovered work so well.[31] By roughly the 1970s, the major 'easy wins' in modern medicine had been played out, and the numbers of lives saved became proportionately fewer despite ever greater investment in drugs and surgery. Indeed, only around half of the seven-year increase in life expectancy gained between 1950 and the end of the century is thought to be attributable to medical interventions, despite the soaring cost. Diminishing returns again.

More recently still, technology has made it possible to save ever more premature babies, and to prolong the lives of ever more decrepit oldies, adding a couple more years in the sun to the average life span. But technology is expensive, and beware those diminishing returns! Despite the billions poured into finding a cure for cancer, exploring genetics or research into lifestyles, pollution and diet, relatively few new remedies have emerged.[32]

Figure 5   Staying alive: life expectancy over time (selected nations)

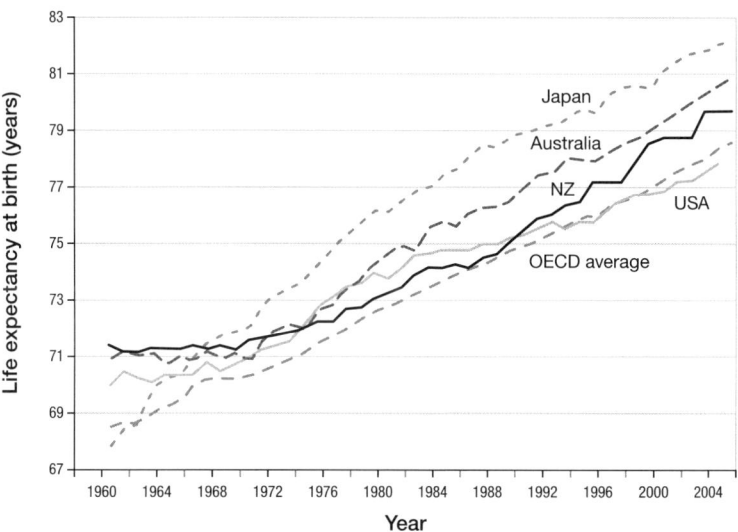

Source   OECD Fact Book 2008

Still, if you look at what's been achieved over the sixty-odd years that modern medicine has been with us, it's hard not to get the impression that the longer you live, the longer you can hope to live. Medicine is producing more and better ways to cure what ails you and to prolong your life for every day you manage to hang in there. Perhaps those crackpots who get themselves snap-frozen against the day medicine discovers a cure for their terminal condition (along with a survivable thawing-out process) aren't so deluded after all. But expert opinion is divided on how long we can keep pushing life expectancy out. Some believe there are natural limits to the human life span. Others say the limit will one day be what we choose it to be. There's even a school of unsettling opinion that points to the current obesity 'epidemic' and warns that we may soon see the perpetual rise in life expectancy reversed.

Looking at the graph, the news is all good, isn't it? New Zealand has a nice, healthy upward-sloping line for life expectancy. People born today should live longer than people ever have in our history, so long as they lay off the greasy burgers and fizzy drinks. New Zealanders' life expectancy at birth is higher than that for the average person in the OECD.

And certainly, if you're of European descent and living in New Zealand, then congratulations – you already have one of the highest life expectancies in the world. You can have about a year more on your life expectancy than the average New Zealander. This means your life expectancy is about the same as people in the elite group of healthy countries, including Australia and Scandinavia. In fact, there are only three countries where blokes live longer than Kiwi European men.

And women live longer than men. On average the difference is four years, which is about 5% extra life, or an extra day of life for every three weeks. Men, with their reckless habits and dodgy Y chromosome, die younger across the board. Even once they've reached the retirement age of 65, a woman can still expect to live two and a half years longer than a man of the same age. Given most women are two years younger than their husbands, this means the average female pensioner can expect four and a half years of peace and quiet at the end of their life. Now that's got to make up for the gender gap in incomes, doesn't it?

Over the last 55 years, the gap between the life expectancies of men and women has widened and then narrowed again, peaking at about six and a half years in the late 1970s. The rise of effective treatment for heart disease has been a major factor in shrinking the gap. Overall, the gap in life expectancy between the sexes is about the same now as it was in 1950 – four years.

Generally, because of the nature of the innovations in medicine, it's the oldies who have seen the biggest proportionate increase in their life expectancy over the past 50 years – particularly women. Non-Maori over 65 have seen their life expectancy extend by 40%, and for those over 90 the improvement has topped 50%. This is consistent with overseas evidence that the investments made in modern medicine since World War Two have tended to benefit the elderly.

Figure 6   **Who has gained from modern medicine?**

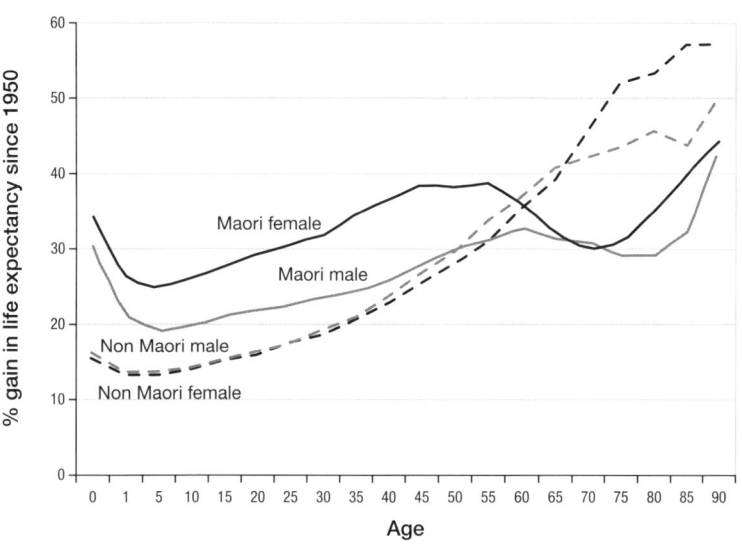

Source   Statistics NZ, Infometrics

So much for all the good stuff about life expectancy. It's time we looked a little more closely.

In 1960, New Zealanders were one of the longest living

bunches of people on the planet. We've since been overtaken by several countries, including Australia and Japan. During that time, our ranking has slipped from 7th to 11th in the OECD. And according to the OECD, we should be doing even worse than that. They've crunched the numbers, considering our risk factors – including, notably, our relatively low health expenditure – and they reckon we should be 0.8 of a year below the average. The fact that we're 1.5 years *better off* than the OECD average baffles everyone.[33] Perhaps we're god's own country after all – good tucker, a benign climate and plenty of exercise from all that chasing sheep around.

Since, as we've seen, we spend less on healthcare in absolute terms, the fact that we're above average in life expectancy means we look pretty efficient when it comes to procuring extra years of life by buying healthcare. That is, we run an effective healthcare system on the smell of an oily rag.

That efficiency has fluctuated over time. We were slightly above-average performers in the late 1960s, when we enjoyed high life expectancy and yet poured just average amounts into the health system. This steadily deteriorated into the 1980s, as funding increased and life expectancy failed to keep pace. It improved again in the wake of the reforms of the late 1980s and early 1990s, as cuts were made to funding. But since the money tap has been turned on again and we continue our slow drift down the life expectancy tables, our efficiency has slipped, too.

Other ways of looking at our life expectancy statistics yield similar news. The OECD drills down to look at how many potential life years are lost by those who die under 70 years of age. The statistics are looking at those people who die younger than the OECD average and counting up the years they would have enjoyed if they'd made the average; needless to say, the more potential years of life lost, the worse your health system looks. In 1960, we were 7th on the OECD table. By 2004, we had dropped to 18th. The actual numbers are (roughly) 9000 years in 1960, and 4000 years in 2004.

Another study eliminates all those deaths that they consider to be 'untreatable'. The rates of these don't change, regardless of how much money you shovel into the health system. These (controversially) include deaths due to accident and suicide, but the idea is to measure the performance of the healthcare system rather than the kind of wider social (and even legal) systems that prevent such tragedies as accidents and suicide. 'Treatable' deaths have declined four times faster than untreatable deaths, and the fall in treatable deaths is roughly proportionate to the rate of healthcare spending (although for some mysterious reason, there seems to be a ten-year lag between spending the money and seeing the result in life expectancy improvements!).[34] But we have been less effective than other OECD nations in getting the rate of treatable deaths down, and unsettlingly, the difference seems to mirror the shortfall in our health spending.

So who's missing out on all those years?

Suffer the children

Most of the money that goes on healthcare in the average lifetime gets spent at the beginning and at the end of life. Obviously, when we're talking about lost potential life years, we're not concerned with the old fogies (who've had a good innings and, for the most part, exceeded the OECD average). Children, on the other hand, stand to lose a great deal if their health needs are not being met. This is one of the areas where things are not looking pretty. Our status as one of the best places in the world to bring up kids is increasingly under question.

In the 1960s, we had the 9th lowest infant mortality rate in the OECD (to be unlucky enough to trouble the scorers in the infant mortality stakes, you have to die under the age of one). By 2005, we had dropped to 21st. This is not quite as bad as it sounds: all of the OECD countries have low levels of infant mortality, so the difference between the top and bottom performers is pretty small. For every 1,000 live births today, we lose between four and seven littlies, which is way better than the 20-35 of fifty years ago.

Figure 7   Infant mortality – selected nations

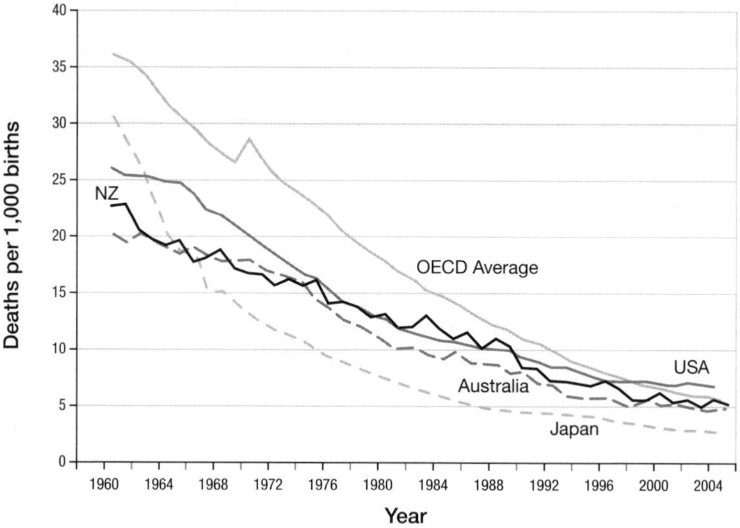

Source   OECD

When you look at the graph above, the first thing that you notice is that everyone is doing better at seeing their infants through that first year of life than they were. But you also notice that we have not been quite as good at it as other nations, and our performance in this regard has slipped from excellent in 1960 to average in 2006.

That's probably why in 2007, UNICEF rated New Zealand amongst the worst of the developed nations for child health, alongside the USA. And it's not so much how many lives we're losing as how we're losing them. The Child Health Index looks at birth weight (where we are average), immunisation rates (our rates have fallen over time and we're now below average) and death rates from accidents and injuries. It's in this last area where we particularly stick out, with a death rate *three times* that of Sweden. This number chimes unpleasantly with the rash of child abuse cases we've seen in the media over the last decade, and it's hard to look at the following graph and feel we do enough to keep our young people safe.

Figure 8   Deaths of under 19 year olds from accidents and injuries

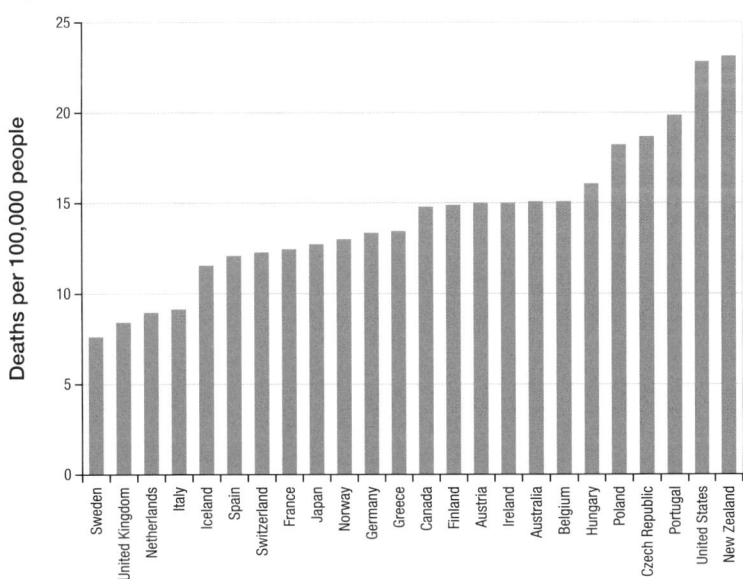

Source   UNICEF

The other groups that miss out on potential years of life are Maori and Pacific Islanders, especially Maori. Since 1950, Maori life expectancy has risen by a third, but a great deal of the catch-up has come from rapidly falling infant mortality, as Figure 9 shows.

These gains are likely to reflect the effect of the kind of basic measures that European New Zealanders had benefited from the better part of 100 years before: sanitation, nutrition, better housing and the prevention of infectious diseases.

Since records began, Maori life expectancy has always been

lower than that of Europeans. Maori men still live eight fewer years than non-Maori men, and Maori women live seven fewer years than non-Maori women. Generally, Maori have been catching up in terms of life expectancy, and Otago University researchers have shown that the gap between Maori and Europeans in death rates for those aged from one to 74 is no longer getting wider: that's progress![35] But while there's any kind of gap at all, there's work to be done.

Figure 9   Infant mortality by ethnicity

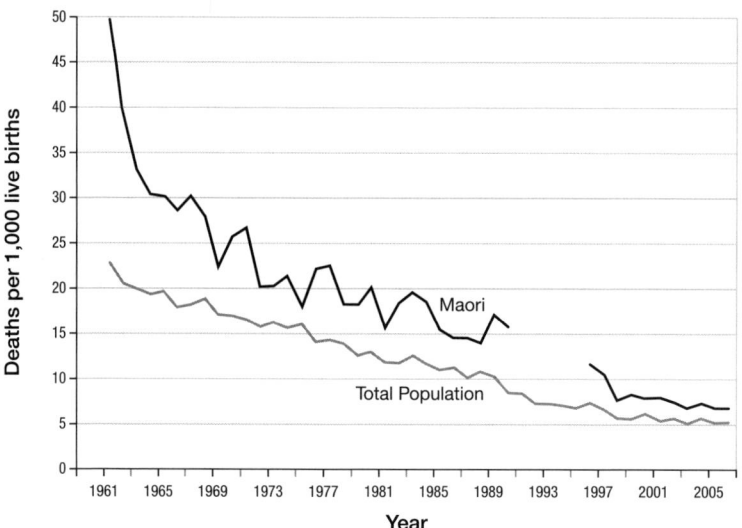

Source   Statistics NZ

So why do Maori live shorter lives? We'll look at this in more detail shortly, and some of the answers will emerge in the discussion of our risk factors and major illnesses, but suffice to say here that the graph below gives a clue: there was a blip in the upward trend in Maori life expectancy, and it coincides with the economic upheaval of the late 80s and early 90s.[36] As we shall see, many things other than the healthcare system have an impact on health. Poverty and unemployment are two such factors, and Maori as a group were worst hit by the economic 'reforms' of that period.

Figure 10 **Mind the gap: life expectancy by ethnicity and gender**

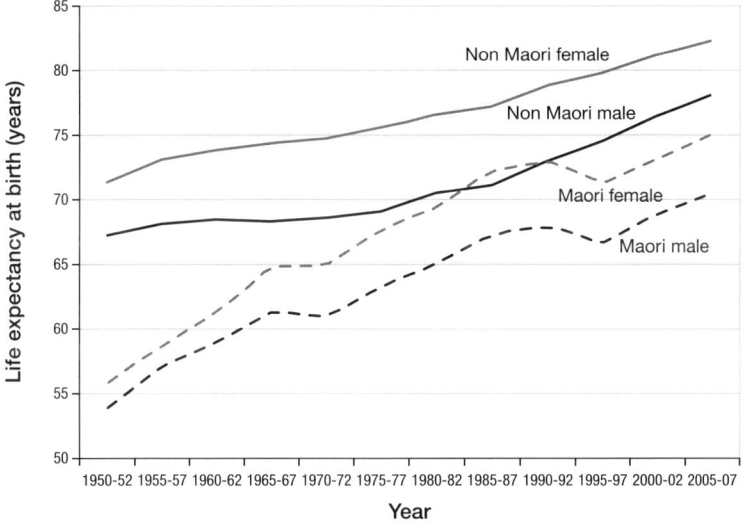

Source   Statistics NZ

After Roger Douglas and Ruth Richardson had done their worst, normal transmission resumed, and the gap narrowed further. But if Maori enjoyed the same life expectancy as non-Maori, New Zealand would be the 6th longest-lived nationality in the OECD rather than the 11th.

We now know how long we live. So what stops us living longer? What are our 'risk indicators' – the behaviours we indulge in that potentially shorten our lives (and if eliminated, potentially prolong them)?

And what, generally speaking, kills us?

Risky business

Smoking

Reductions in smoking rates have been nothing short of dramatic. With only 22% of the population still in thrall to the gaspers, we are now near the lowest in the OECD for smoking rates, particularly for men. Given that one in two smokers will lose 15 years of their life to a smoking-related illness, this is a big deal.[37] New Zealand men and women now have very similar rates of smoking. This is unusual – overseas women tend to smoke less than men. The equality of the sexes can be taken too far.

Still, New Zealand loses the equivalent of a town the size of Ngaruawahia (5000 people) each year to smoking-related deaths,[38] and the statistics indicate that the population of that town, like the population of the real-life Ngaruawahia, is overwhelmingly Maori. Smoking rates among Maori are still almost *double* – around 44% of the Maori population smoke. This is clearly one contributor to the dire Maori health statistics we've touched upon.[39]

Reducing smoking is one of the most cost-effective methods to improve national health,[40] and it's important, for this reason, that we press on with the hard work that has gone into tobacco control in recent years, particularly among Maori.

Figure 11 **Stubbing it out: smoking rates over time**

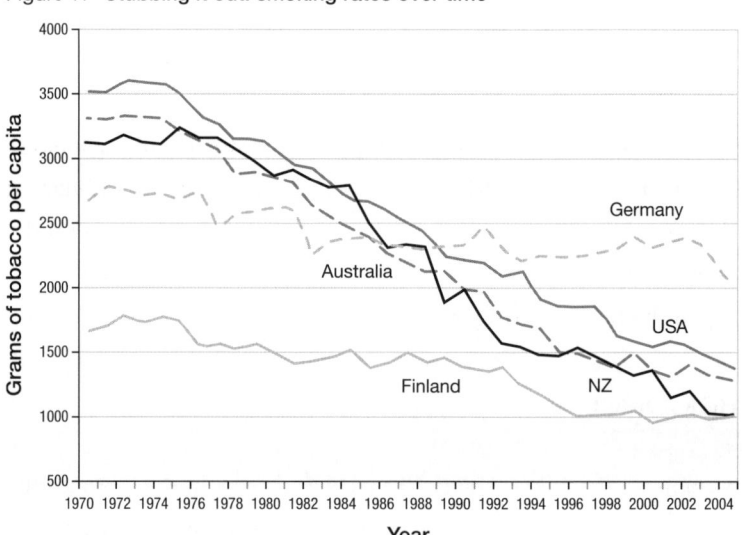

Source   OECD Health Data 2008

Smoking can also inflict collateral damage through second-hand smoke exposure. One in 10 children and one in 13 adult non-smokers are exposed to second-hand smoke in their home. Once again, the worst hit are children growing up in poor communities, particularly where smoking is prevalent – that is, among Maori.

Gotcha – to give up

Len used to smoke only when he had a drink, or when he took his horses to the races. Since his wife died he smoked more and more frequently. Like most men in his seventies, Len eventually needed a hip operation. His GP told him he wouldn't get his operation so long as he was smoking. Len duly gave up smoking that day, and didn't touch a cigarette until he got his operation.

While recuperating from his operation, he noticed that other patients were going outside for a smoke. He made enquiries, and found out that the supposed restriction didn't exist at all – his doctor was having him on. But the cunning ruse worked: Len still isn't smoking to this day. Should we have a restriction like this? The state – which picks up after us as we indulge in our risky behaviours – has the power to demand you adopt a healthy lifestyle or your access to public health services will be limited. It's worth a thought.

Alcohol

Total alcohol consumption has also fallen, and New Zealand now knocks back something close to the OECD average of the strong stuff. The vast majority of New Zealanders drink alcohol, right across the age spectrum. In fact, three out of four people aged 15 to 17 admit they've had an alcoholic drink in the past year, even though by law they aren't supposed to. But to paraphrase a recent advertising campaign, it's not how much we're drinking, but how we're drinking. In 2006/2007, about a quarter of drinkers aged 15 years and over had a potentially hazardous drinking pattern, with over half of young men aged 18-24 having what the Ministry of Health calls a 'dangerous drinking pattern'. So what's a 'dangerous drinking pattern' then – drinking Flaming Sambuccas while wearing a nylon shirt, or having a beer while sitting on the roof? In fact, it's about binge drinking – sitting down with a bunch of drink and deliberately setting about getting drunk. Binging is a national pastime, and binge drinkers can be found in all sectors of New Zealand society – from poor to wealthy, and women as well as men. Needless to say, dangerous drinking is also relatively high amongst Maori and Pacific Island communities.[41]

Diet and obesity

There's a common saying that when someone gives up smoking, they get fat instead. Well, nicotine does suppress appetite. And we've seen that New Zealand has been pretty good at swearing off tobacco as a nation: national statistics suggest that as we've turned away from cigarettes, we've turned to steak and cheese pies instead. The rate of obesity has risen from one in 10 adults in 1977 to one in four now. It's one of our most highly visible problems.

To determine healthy (and unhealthy) body weights, a crude calculation called the body mass index (BMI) is used. This is derived by dividing your weight in kilograms by the number you get when you square your height in metres. For adults aged 18 years and over, you're considered 'obese' if your BMI is greater than or equal to 30 kg/m^2. So if you're the average Kiwi male height of 1.77 metres, 94 kgs is your obesity threshold. If you're the average female height of 1.64 metres,[42] you should aim to be under 81kg.

If you're crunching the numbers and fretting because you're falling foul of them, you needn't necessarily panic. The lines are pretty arbitrary, and have no regard for body shape, fitness or ethnic grouping, all of which can mean a few extra kilos are neither here nor there from a health perspective. Piri Weepu and Richie McCaw of the 2009 All Blacks, for example, are both borderline obese according to their BMI. There's less doubt about Ma'a Nonu and most of the squad's front row, all of whom BMI pronounces obese. Perhaps that's why we lost the Tri-Nations trophy this year!

With this caveat in mind, let's look at the facts. New Zealand is now among the top quarter of OECD nations for levels of obesity.

Figure 12 **Heavyweight contenders: obesity rates by country**

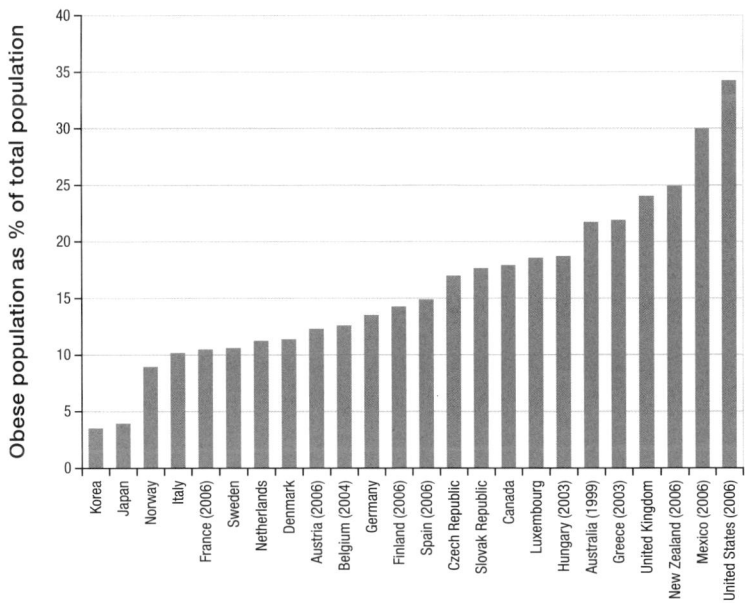

Sources OECD Health Data (2008) & Ministry of Social Development Social Report (2008) –
all figures 2005 unless stated

Around 12% of Asians, 23% of European/Other, 43% of Maori and a whopping 65% of Pacific Island people are considered obese. This may be due to the different body types (or sporting habits) of ethnic groups, and an artefact of the rather crude measure that is used to determine obesity. But this quibbling is unlikely to explain away the issue altogether.

Despite the fears often expressed about the amount of biomass you see in primary school playgrounds, the rate of childhood obesity seems to have peaked at around 8% for boys and 9% for girls, and has even shown signs of falling in recent years.[43] Again, though, obesity rates are still significantly higher for Pacific and Maori communities, at 23% and 12% respectively, than for European and Asian children, which lurk around 6%.

Figure 13 **Obesity rates by ethnicity**

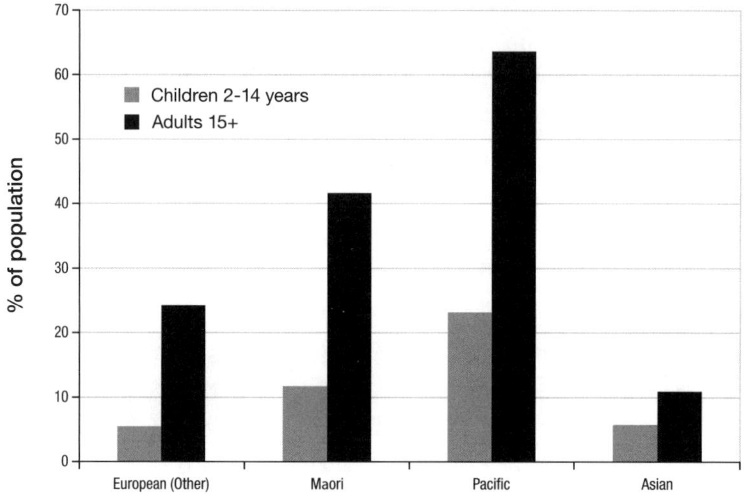

Source   MSD Social Report 2008

And yes, we should care, because obesity is associated with a long list of adult health conditions, including: cardiovascular disease (ischaemic heart disease, high blood pressure and stroke), various types of cancer, type 2 diabetes, kidney disease, fatty liver disease, osteoarthritis, pulmonary embolism, deep vein thrombosis, polycystic ovarian syndrome, gout, gallstones, reproductive disorders, sleep apnoea, complications in pregnancy, complications in surgery, and psychological and social problems.[44] The nightmare scenario with obesity is that it leads to increased levels of diabetes, and in turn diabetes leads to all sorts of other 'co-morbidities'. In other words, overweight people tend to develop other conditions, too. All those fatties could very quickly become a heavy burden for the health system.

While we're seeing some evidence of this, the rise in diabetes complications thankfully hasn't mirrored the rise in obesity. Have we got off lightly, or is the worst yet to come? No one knows.

We noted above that fears had been raised that the 'obesity epidemic' could see the present, corpulent generation reverse the trend of life expectancies that has been on an upward march since Victorian times. Luckily, though, the link between obesity and certain, premature death is not so straightforward as all that. Obesity is merely a risk factor among other risk factors, such as hypertension, smoking and high cholesterol intake. Thankfully, it seems that on a national scale, at least, the increased health problems arising from obesity will not be significant enough to offset the substantial benefits arising from reductions in smoking. There are also some tentative signs that the growth in the rate of obesity is slowing and may even have stopped altogether. There has been no significant increase in obesity levels amongst both young people and adults since 2002.[45]

Dr Morgan's miracle diet

Deteriorating diet is a major driver behind the growth in obesity, and clearly a balanced diet and sensible exercise regime are among the best things you can do for your health.

So what constitutes a balanced diet? There is less than 100% scientific consensus on the best diet to keep you lean and mean. Each camp has its theory, and other camps all have conspiracy theories about those theories. Some experts argue that animal-sourced 'saturated' fat increases the levels of 'bad' cholesterol in our blood, which blocks our arteries and causes heart disease. A closely related argument is that the human body struggles to deal with animal-sourced proteins like meat and dairy, resulting in diseases like cancer.

Opponents of this kind of talk argue that this is all scaremongering perpetrated by the drug companies, who want the population to live in fear so that they can sell us cholesterol-lowering drugs.

Other experts argue that the growth in carbohydrate consumption is to blame for obesity and its associated woes. They argue that the modern Western diet is calorie-rich, and nutrient-poor, and that once we eat more calories than we use, we tend to get fatter because we store that excess energy. This is especially the case for saturated fats and refined carbohydrates, like white flour and sugar. Their opponents argue these experts are the stooges of the meat and dairy industries.

Yet more experts claim that diet doesn't make much of a difference to our health at all, and that the human body is fairly tolerant of what it eats. Studies have been undertaken on the impact of diet on heart disease to test whether a 'Mediterranean diet' or 'Japanese lifestyle' would help reduce Western cholesterol levels and subsequently reduce heart attacks. They can have an impact, but it doesn't seem to be that significant. While cholesterol is certainly a risk factor for heart disease, patients had to reduce the amount of cholesterol eaten by 25% to reduce cholesterol levels in the blood by 5%.[46] Diet helps, but the body naturally regulates things quite well. Other factors may be partly to blame for our modern health problems. Indeed, it's even been suggested that it may have been a bacterium like chlamydia that triggered the real epidemic of heart disease in the 1970s! Certainly diet alone can't have caused the huge rise in heart disease – our consumption of fat hardly budged when heart attacks shot up by 50%. And it's not as though we've sworn off greasy burgers since then, yet heart attack rates have receded again. Recent research has shown the flu may play a role in triggering heart attacks. Genetics may also determine what the effect of different diets may have. New Zealand Asians have the lowest rates of fruit and vegetable intake and exercise in the population, but they also have the lowest rates of obesity. That's why diet is a risk factor rather than a health denominator. You can't always predict a bad outcome from a crook diet, any more than you can say for certain that smoking will carry you away to a premature grave. Talk to any smoker, and you will eventually hear an anecdote of how they met someone who smoked 20 a day and still lived to see their 100th birthday. Conversely, everyone seems to have a friend of a friend who ran 10 kilometres a day, drank in moderation and ate healthily only to drop dead or enter the cancer ward at 40.

In short, the links between exercise, what you eat and your health are incredibly complex. It is very difficult for science to isolate 'causes' because so much depends upon other factors, combinations of foods and what is substituted when a food gets cut from a person's diet.

For example, the recent focus on reducing saturated fat intake was a good thing, but it has pushed food manufacturers to increase sugar and salt levels in order to compensate for the loss in taste. And so we now have a plethora of 99% fat free foods, which are crammed with sugar and salt instead. This doesn't help in the quest for health. Nor is it likely to help if sugar and salt are displaced by yet another cocktail of other chemicals whose long-term effects are untested – such as the artificial sweetener aspartame, and monosodium glutamate.

So where does that leave us? As usual with such debates, everyone is probably a little bit right. So sorry, folks. You'll have to find a diet that works for you, because the medical world doesn't have a silver bullet. Still, there are a few things most scientists seem to agree on:

- Eating more calories than we use makes us fatter. If you burn the calories through exercise, then it doesn't matter too much what you eat. That is why our sheep-shearing grandfathers could eat bacon and eggs for breakfast every day and not get fat. But once you don't burn the calories, you put on weight. Excess calories from fat are probably worse for clogging your arteries than those from sugar, but ultimately we either need to reduce calorie intake or exercise more.

- Where you do eat carbohydrate, make it as unprocessed as possible – e.g. brown bread rather than white. The energy in unprocessed carbohydrates gets released into your bloodstream slowly, while processed sugar and flour are dumped on your metabolism all at once. This gives you a temporary sugar hit, but like every drug, it leaves you down and needing more. Fizzy drinks in particular are stacked with sugar – give your teeth a break and stick with good old fluoridated tap water. We will see below that the chief suspect in the growth of New Zealand's obesity has to be increased refined sugar consumption.

- New Zealanders probably eat more meat and dairy produce than is ideal for their long-term health – these vices are probably one factor in our high rates of heart disease and colon cancer.[47]

- Eat plenty of fruit and vegetables – five servings a day is a minimum, not an aspiration. Wherever possible, eat them unprocessed and raw – over-cooking can often destroy the nutrients. If you like a bit of heat, quickly steam them rather than boiling. Microwaving turns food into nutritionally valueless mush.

It's one of the marvels of nature that the differing colours of fruit and veges are good signifiers of different nutrients, so go for bright colours and mix them up as much as possible.

- A good rule of thumb is the more you see a food advertised, the less you should eat it. If it's advertised – even if it advertises health benefits – it's processed, and if it's processed, it's probably lost most of its nutritional value.[48] In the words of Michael Pollan: 'Eat food. Not too much, mostly plants.'[49]

The figures on food consumption themselves are quite surprising.[50] The image of New Zealand as a mutton-chomping, dairy-glutted nation is somewhat questionable these days. We eat less protein and fat than the rest of the OECD, whereas the reverse was true in 1960. This is not altogether because we're eating less of these things: mostly it's because the rest of the OECD is eating more. We eat more fruit and vegetables than the international average, and our intake has been growing faster than the average. However, our vegetable intake has been falling in recent years in favour of a rise in fruit consumption.[51] The real surprise comes on sugar intake. New Zealanders consume a third more sugar than people in rich nations overseas. Sugar intake has been rising rapidly across the OECD in the past forty years, and New Zealand is emphatically no exception.

So all-in-all, the culprits in the rising rates of obesity are not hard to find. Sugar consumption is up, and is higher than overseas. One in five children has three or more fizzy drinks every week, and the same number has fast food at least twice a week. Exercise rates are falling, although slowly. Two out of three children watch two or more hours of television every day.[52] Again, the main problems are among Maori and Pacific Island communities, and amongst the poor. Perhaps it's time to ban the drinks machine and bring back milk in schools?

Other factors

Some surprising things seem to have an effect on the health of different groups in society, if their correlation with poor health statistics is anything to go by.[53] Studies have shown that income, inequality of income distribution (or 'status' in society), the level and kind of social contact you enjoy, the extent of female education, level of ethnic fragmentation, and even predominant religion all seem to play a role in health and well-being.[54][55] But the one that really seems to have a big health impact – and the one that seems to account for much of the difference between Pacific Island and Maori communities on the one hand and their better-off Pakeha counterparts on the other – is unemployment.[56] Not only does unemployment reduce income, it also impacts on self-esteem. Some researchers have equated the size of this impact on health to smoking 10 packs of cigarettes a day![57]

Meanwhile, other studies have shown that death rates increase during times of economic boom – when people are doing lots of overtime, or perhaps just getting stressed about what to do with all that income.[58] So it may be that one of the best things the government can do to improve health is not actually to build another hospital, but instead to provide a stable economy with a steady, predictable rate of growth, without too many of those exciting peaks and troughs that seem to take such a toll on us.

Research seems to indicate that there's a link between increased income *inequality* and increased health problems.[59] The argument is that in developed countries, absolute income matters not a jot for your ability to look after yourself. (In the Third World, of course, absolute income has a profound impact on your ability to look after yourself). The impact of being *relatively* poor is thought to be capable of having a dire impact on your stress levels (e.g. from lower self-esteem), your understanding of health issues and could perhaps even reduce your access to essential healthcare. All that bitterness you feel as you wait beside your broken-down Nissan

Cedric while a procession of late-model Beamers cruise past just isn't good for you. If so, this may explain some of the disparities between Pakeha on the one hand and Maori and Pacific Islanders on the other. Does this mean it's time for a Revolution, comrade? Not really, and nor does it even justify hiking taxes on the rich: remember that national income was the most important driver. It's easier to improve equality through Government spending than complicated taxes[60] – another reason to make sure that health spending is helping those who need it most.

Even our relationships play a part in our healthiness. This should be no surprise: our friends and family are a powerful source of purpose and nurturing.[61] Yet these considerations are rarely given much airing in a conversation about our health system.

In short, it's worth repeating the point that we mostly think of the health system as what makes us better when we're ill. But actually, if our aim is improving health standards generally, the correct approach addresses all those aspects of our lives that contribute to keeping us well. And as we've discussed, this sheets back strongly to living conditions and incomes.

Common afflictions

It is also possible to break our deaths down by condition and compare our performance with overseas,[62] and we will focus our attention on the biggest killers overall. A quick word of caution on statistics. At various times you've probably heard that cancer or heart disease or something else is the biggest killer in New Zealand. Depending on how the categories are grouped together or broken down, the top killer can be very different. Between deaths from all types of cancer, heart disease and strokes, it's possible to account for 2/3 of all deaths in New Zealand.

Cancer

Cancer deaths are the biggest killer overall, and mortality

is fairly evenly distributed between lung, breast, colon, and prostate cancer.

Overall, New Zealand does slightly worse than the rest of the OECD in terms of cancer rates. The most noticeable issue is colon cancer rates, which seem to be around 50% higher than the OECD average. Think about that next time you decide to have burnt bacon instead of All Bran for breakfast. This is balanced a bit by lower lung cancer rates – presumably because of the success we've had in reducing the numbers of people who smoke. Breast, cervical and prostate cancer rates are all slightly above average. Maori cancer death rates are 60% higher than non-Maori rates for men and 80% higher for women.[63]

Heart disease

Heart disease is the second biggest killer overall.

Our death rate from heart disease is a particular area of concern, both in terms of the absolute number of deaths and in terms of how it compares internationally. New Zealanders have a 30% higher chance of dying from a heart attack than the average OECD citizen. Maori are even worse off, with around an 80% higher chance of dying than a Pakeha. Many people point to our high intake of saturated (basically animal) fat – Kiwis get through 27 litres of ice cream per person each year, compared with Australians at 17.8 litres.[64] This could be one reason why heart disease has us licked! The rate at which people developed cholesterol levels that require medication are particularly high for Asian men and Pacific Island women, and heart disease seems significantly higher for Maori and Pacific Island women than their European counterparts.[65]

Strokes

Strokes most commonly occur when objects – usually blood clots, or chunks of the gunk that clogs arteries – lodge in the brain and do damage. They are usually caused by hypertension (high blood pressure). New Zealand is famous for its laid-back attitude, and this must have some impact on our blood pressure, because while it's still a big killer, our rate of strokes is below the OECD average. This is particularly the case for Kiwi men. She'll be right, mate!

Respiratory diseases

These are another big ticket killer, and most of the deaths are related to smoking. As you'd expect given our low smoking rates, New Zealand does fairly well in these stakes. This is no cause to ease off, though: getting the diehard smokers to quit is so cost-effective a way to improve health across the board that it makes perfect sense to keep up the pressure.

New Zealand seems to make an excellent fist of preventing deaths from influenza, bronchitis and pneumonia, but it's let down somewhat by the high prevalence of asthma. As we shall see later on, we could do a lot better at treating asthma, too. Respiratory illnesses are more of a problem for Maori and women in deprived communities.[66]

'External' causes

Remarkably, given all the press coverage crime and accidents receive, 'external' causes of death (anything unrelated to what is considered a 'medical condition') only account for 7% of our mortality. Only two in every 1000 Kiwis die from violent crime, contrary to the impression you'd get from the newspapers and from the bleatings of the Sensible Sentencing Trust. The two major players here are car crashes and suicide. More on suicide below. Road deaths are 16% higher than the OECD average – in particular, death rates for females are higher than their overseas counterparts. The clear message is ease off the gas, girls!

Mental health

While not a big cause of death in its own right, mental health has a huge impact on quality of life, and when suicide is taken into account, it becomes an important issue. As shown in the chart below, New Zealand has high rates of poor mental health, and this is filtering through into higher death rates. This is another issue to watch for the future, as mental health problems are increasing rapidly (whether because more of us are losing it, or because we're braver about admitting it or better at diagnosing it is unclear). Interestingly, Europeans have higher rates of officially diagnosed mental illness, but there's some evidence that Maori and Pacific Islanders may be suffering with high rates of mental illness that goes undetected or at least untreated.

Figure 14 **Mental health problems**

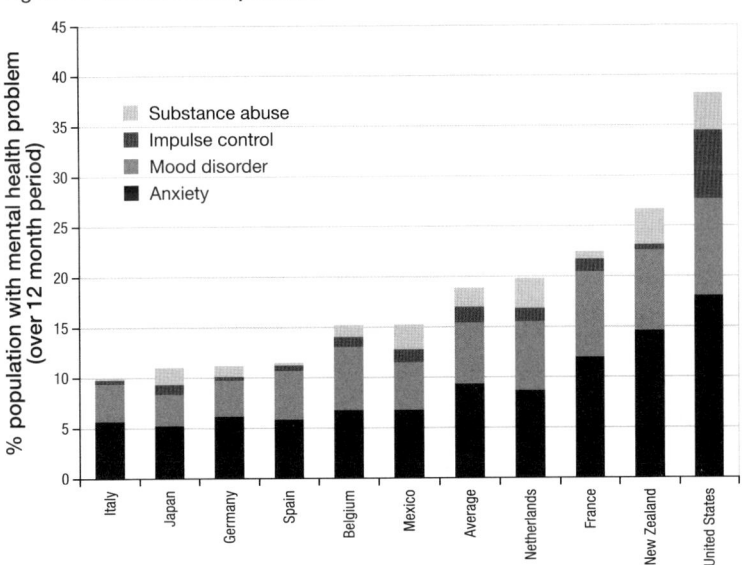

Source   OECD Social Indicators 2009

Hormonal and nutritional diseases
We are slightly above average for deaths from hormonal and nutritional diseases such as diabetes. All the same, death rates are relatively low for these conditions. This may be partly due to the fact that diabetes is often related to other problems, such as heart disease. Given the rise in obesity, these conditions need to be watched carefully. Already the warning signs are appearing in the Maori population, where deaths from diabetes mellitus are *five times* higher than for the general population.[67] Although this is starting from a low base, this is a concern for the future.

Loose ends
We do well in controlling infectious diseases generally. AIDS is well under control, compared to other countries. The dental health of our children is quite good, thanks to public coverage until age 18 and the fluoridation of water supplies in our major population centres. Above the age of 18, however, dental problems seem to be another particular issue for Maori and Pacific Island communities.

We also do exceptionally well with low deaths from cirrhosis of the liver — let's drink to that!

Death vs disability
One final point is that the rankings above are based on what kills us. If you also take into account *disability* caused by various conditions, things look a bit different. In particular, mental health issues rise to prominence, because even if they don't kill large numbers of us, they do have a huge impact on our well-being.

The table opposite sets out the top ten conditions ranked by their impact on disability length of life.

Top ten conditions by impact on disability and lost life	
Heart disease	13%
Stroke	5.4%
Chronic obstructive respiratory disease	4.9%
Diabetes	3.8%
Depression	3.6%
Asthma	3.3%
Anxiety	3.2%
Lung cancer	3.2%
Road traffic	3.1%
Colo-rectal cancer	2.9%

Source Ministry of Health (2001), *The Burden of Disease and Injury in New Zealand*

So in sum, we have done well to reduce smoking, but perhaps to help with our nicotine withdrawal we've turned to the cakes instead – obesity is high. In terms of major conditions, cancer and heart disease are the big killers. Compared to overseas however, the areas that stand out most are heart disease, colon cancer and road deaths. Much work has already taken place on these issues, but more is clearly needed. So despite the rapid fall in heart disease, it remains probably the biggest challenge for the New Zealand health system.

Quality of life

So much for all the statistics that tell us how long we live, and what kills us when we stop. They don't tell us much about our quality of life. Who knows, we might all be spending our four-score years moping about afflicted by all manner of illnesses that manage to make our lives misery without ever quite ending them. And with our doctors getting better and better at keeping us alive when we're on the way out, we might be spending a disproportionate amount of time rigged up to machines in the hush of a hospital ward, waiting for the flick of the switch.

Thankfully there isn't much evidence that we suffer from either nightmare scenario – New Zealanders are about average for 'healthy lifespan' (the number of years lived without disability)[68] – and our healthy lifespan also seems to be increasing along with our life expectancy.[69] People are remaining active for longer, and we seem to incur the bulk of our life's healthcare bills in the last couple of years of life. In the healthcare business, this is called the *compression of morbidity*, just in case you want to look smart at your next cocktail party. A reduced proportion of elderly people living out their days in a state of disability also shrinks the average costs of caring for an elderly person. So this is good news – you should be able to keep on motorcycling until that last ride, where Parkinson's suddenly descends and you shake off a bend. When the end comes, let's hope for all our sakes – for the victim and the taxpayer – it comes quick.

How healthy do we feel?

So the stats say we're living longer, healthier lives than ever before. Why, then, the vast 'Health' section in the bookshops, the raft of ads on prime-time TV peddling drugs and supplements to give you a boost?

Despite the relentless march of modern healthcare, the average citizen of the modern world is generally less satisfied with their health than they were 25 years ago. The first world has more sick days and registers more episodes of ill health than previous generations.[70] Collectively we go to the GP more, yet the vast majority (one study suggests 85%) of these visits are not associated with any diagnosable condition.[71]

Why is this? Researchers have suggested a number of reasons. First, disease used to kill us off pretty quick, probably before we'd had much time to think about it. After all, when you're young and fit, nothing can touch you. Now, however, we've treated the diseases that used to knock off the young and complacent, and we're left with chronic, lingering diseases like diabetes, asthma and heart disease. Mortality is brought more sharply into the collective consciousness of an ageing population, hence the burgeoning 'health industry'. And perhaps most importantly, the very success of medicine has created heightened expectations that anything can be cured. Whereas in the past, our pioneer forebears would have bit the bullet and worked through the pain, we now think we're entitled to duvet days and as much pain relief as we can swallow until the problem is sorted. Sadly, doctors are not miracle workers and most people eventually get disappointed.

Nonetheless, in a world where everyone feels a little poorly, New Zealanders are far and away the most contented with their state of health.[72] We rate highly on many international surveys of happiness and well-being. This would be a cause for some celebration, were it not for the fact that the United States, which suffers from all manner of dysfunctions according to the stats that mean anything, is a close second. Perhaps they should screen their survey respondents to exclude people on Prozac.

Scoring our health system

Overall international comparison
There is no one fact or figure that you can point to in order to give our health system a pass or fail on its effectiveness, or even the bang we get for our buck. However, there is one reasonably comprehensive international survey (undertaken by the Commonwealth Fund) that covers the inputs, outputs (adjusted for quality) and outcomes of the health systems of six Western countries. It has the advantage of addressing important aspects of healthcare not captured by stark vital statistics. These parts make for interesting reading:
• Access: largely thanks to the private sector network of GPs,

New Zealanders have no problem accessing basic healthcare. The only problem seems to be the cost of co-payments: for people on lower incomes, that $30 consultation fee is pretty steep (although there's evidence to suggest this cost barrier has reduced since the survey was last taken).

- Patient Safety: we're about average. Reported hospital complications are currently on the rise in New Zealand, but it's likely that this says more about how much tidier we've got in our reporting procedures than how ragged our hospitals are getting.

- Coordination: New Zealand GPs have comparatively advanced IT systems that facilitate coordination between the various services and sectors within the system as a whole. Given the number of medical errors that nevertheless arise from the lack of an effective patient handover, and the cases we've found of people getting 'lost' in the system, there's clearly work to be done on improving links (both informal and IT-based) between GPs and hospitals. In fact, anecdotally, hospital systems often even cannot coordinate across different specialities. This is a big deal, because many patients have more than one problem and end up getting bumped from pillar to post. But we rank highly in coordination compared to many countries: one can only wonder what it's like overseas!

- Patient-Centred-ness: New Zealand does pretty well on this measure, too, and there has been a vast and concerted effort to change the culture of our health providers since the 1970s, when the so-called 'unfortunate experiment' at National Women's Hospital highlighted what can happen when the system is all about the doctors. Still, we came across several examples where the attitude of medical staff to a patient has been counterproductive. There's always a need for constant vigilance and continuous improvement in this area. As we shall see, there's particular room for improvement on how the health system deals with different cultures, and also deals with innovative new ways of staying in touch with patients.

- Correct care: There are some questions over whether the 'right' care is always delivered. This may suggest the need for ways to keep frontline doctors up to date with medical developments, and to ensure key conditions are treated according to clinical best practice.
- Patient/Doctor Satisfaction: these are both similar to other countries.

Overall, the last iteration of this survey gave New Zealand a solid 'C' mark – not failing, but not top of the class either.

The main concern here is that a few years ago New Zealand was top of the class. Since 2004, we've been overtaken by all but Canada and the US. This may be partly due to the rather rigorous performance management systems that have been put in place in other countries over recent years.

Summary

So what have we learned? All-in-all, we do pretty well given how much we spend (and can afford to spend) on health. New Zealanders do pretty well in terms of lifespan – and presumably this is what we are most interested in – although our advantage has been slipping. Our success is only partly the result of our efficient health system; it could be that it's at least partly due to living in godzone. Our health system actually churns out fewer operations than overseas. This is a result of spending less on healthcare, which is because we are a relatively poor nation in OECD terms. So if we want better healthcare – or at least a health system with more outputs and some improvement in outcomes – we should really focus on getting richer. Quickly.

Finally, what have we learned about the returns from investing in healthcare? Based on recent increases, if you put more money into your healthcare system, it's unlikely that you will get the same increase in hospital activity, let alone health outcomes. In fact, based on the information we've seen so far, if we doubled

Ranking (out of 6)	Australia	Canada	Germany	New Zealand	United Kingdon	United States
Overall Ranking (2007)	3.5	5	2	3.5	1	6
Overall Care	4	6	2.5	2.5	1	5
Right Care	5	6	3	4	2	1
Safe Care	4	5	1	3	2	6
Coordinated Care	3	6	4	2	1	5
Patient-Centered Care	3	6	2	1	4	5
Access	3	5	1	2	4	6
Efficiency	4	5	3	2	1	6
Equity	2	5	4	3	1	6
Long, Healthy, and Productive Lives	1	3	2	4.5	4.5	6
Health Expenditures per Capita, 2004	**$2,876***	**$3,165**	**$3,005***	**$2,083**	**$2,546**	**$6,102**

Source: Commonwealth Fund 2007

Overall Rankings

	Australia	Canada	Germany	New Zealand	United Kingdon	United States
Overall Ranking (2007 Edition)	3.5	5	2	3.5	1	6
Overall Ranking (2006 Edition)	4	5	1	2	3	6
Overall Ranking (2004 Edition)	2	4	n/a	1	3	6
Health Expenditures per Capita, 2004	$2,876*	$3,165	$3,005*	$2,083	$2,546	$6,102

Source Commonwealth Fund 2007

our health budget (to 18% of our national income), it seems likely we would get about a 30% increase in the number of operations, and perhaps an additional two years of average life expectancy. This is about a 3% increase in your lifespan – from 79.6 years to around 82 years. Sure, this would put us within reach of the very top countries in the world in terms of life expectancy. But it would come at an enormous cost. Incredibly, we could as a nation get roughly the same health benefits at very little cost if everyone stopped smoking, exercised and improved their diet.[73] But will we give up our beer and pizza now to live another two to three years later on in life? Fat chance.

Until we can see exactly what we get when we put more money into the health system (the answer so far seems to be better paid staff rather than more staff or more productivity), there has to be a serious question mark over whether we simply keep on shovelling more and more money into the system.

A big concern has to be obesity. While the long-term health implications may not be as apocalyptic as some predict, this trend will definitely impact on our health system. We're already seeing a harbinger of the change in rising diabetes rates. While heart disease rates are falling, it remains a far bigger killer here than overseas. The only unmitigated good news out of the morbidity statistics is that we've lately been very effective at getting smoking rates down, and we're reaping the rewards in the form of reductions in respiratory disease.

But by far the biggest concern is Maori health. Good progress has been made in improving Maori life expectancy – apart from a blip in the 1990s: kia ora, Ruth! – but more effort is needed, both to understand and to address the discrepancy. Quite apart from the fact that this is a significant part of our nation we're letting down, Maori and Pacific peoples are an increasing proportion of the population: their lower life expectancy will become more and more visible in our national statistics in coming years. Logically, a focus on Maori and Pacific health would also be more cost-effective than other areas that might be targeted for spending. Rather than throwing ever more money at old white people – where the marginal returns swiftly diminish – the numbers of Maori who would benefit from relatively simpler investments in public health would be greater per dollar spent. As we shall see in coming chapters, focusing on issues like vaccinations, infant mortality, smoking, obesity, and lower injury rates[74] tend to have very big payoffs in terms of health improvements.

It's certainly no coincidence that Maori and Pacific Islanders tend to be over-represented among the poor, and that the poor have more and more serious health issues than the better off. This is most obscenely evident in the US, where the privileged few receive every piece of healthcare possible, while the poor miss out. Each extra bit of healthcare received by the rich makes a very small difference to when they die (but boy, they die in style), yet the same amount of money would make a huge difference to the lifespan of America's poor. This explains how it is that America spends the most on healthcare of any country in the world, yet on average has some of the worst health outcomes. If we assume every year of life has the same value, then America would be hugely better off spending less on nips and tucks for the rich and more on hips and hearts for the poor. The same applies here, the interventions and treatments needed by Maori are likely to be simpler, cheaper and yield better results.

So finally, then, it may be time to question whether the pendulum of health concerns in New Zealand has swung too far in the direction of the elderly. The elderly, particularly males over 65, have gained the most from the past fifty years of investment in healthcare. Meanwhile, low immunisation rates and high accident rates mean that the health of our young has begun ringing alarm bells in the OECD.

Something, somewhere has gone wrong with the logic of our spending.

Maori health

As we've just seen, European New Zealanders have some of the highest life expectancies in the Western World. The flipside of this is that Maori have among the lowest. These sorts of comparisons are a bit hokey, but on average a Maori male has the same life expectancy as the vodka and sausage-guzzling chaps of Poland and the Slovak Republic. Maori females on the other hand have about the same life expectancy as a Turkish woman. Don't get me wrong, Turkey is a lovely place, but trust me you wouldn't want to get sick there.

The Maori population was knocked sideways by the arrival of the Europeans, who brought with them all sorts of nasty bugs that the Maori had never encountered. No one is quite sure how many Maori were here before the Europeans arrived but estimates vary between 50-80% of the population were killed by infectious diseases. Over time, the Maori population has recovered, and their life expectancy has improved. However, Maori life expectancy has never quite caught up with the life expectancy of Europeans.

This difference in life expectancy is due to a number of things. Income and employment is certainly a factor. Just under 11% of Maori are unemployed, as opposed to 5% of the New Zealand population more generally.[75] As we have already seen unemployment can have a devastating impact on health through its impacts on income and self-esteem. The current economic recession, like the one in the 1990s, is hitting Maori disproportionately hard – their unemployment rate has risen faster than the national average.[76] That this could result in a further setback to their life expectancy seems far-fetched to some of us, but the evidence supports such an outcome.

Income and jobs alone are not enough to explain the difference. Even when income is accounted for, wealthier Maori still have worse outcomes than their wealthier European counterparts.[77] Healthy lifestyles are another factor. As we have seen, rates of smoking and obesity are higher among Maori and Pacific Islanders than other populations. These issues show up in the kinds of illnesses where there are higher rates amongst Maori and Pacific populations, such as chronic obstructive pulmonary (i.e. lung) disease. Maori and Pacific children have lower rates of eating breakfast at home, higher intake of fizzy drinks and fast food and receive more physical punishment.

Maori children also watch more television and are exposed to higher rates of second-hand smoke. As adults, Maori and Pacific Islanders are more likely to gamble, have hazardous drinking patterns and not exercise.[78] Clearly considerable work is needed to improve the lifestyles of Maori and Pacific people if life-spans are to increase. And this data is corrected for income, so it's not to be confused with being a poor person's propensity: these are lifestyle consequences. However, even this is not the full story of the difference in life expectancy.

This brings us to a less acceptable aspect of Maori and Pacific interaction with their health system. Despite a higher prevalence of certain conditions, Maori and Pacific Islanders don't have these conditions diagnosed and treated by the health system. One study even suggested that for Pacific Islanders, the healthcare system had made no contribution to improving their health over the past 25 years.[79] Why?

Getting initial access to the health system is an issue – Maori rates for visiting a GP are slightly lower than for Europeans. More importantly, Maori and Pacific Islanders have double the rates of unmet need – times when they needed to see a GP but were unable to.[80] Partly this is a result of the co-payments we pay in healthcare: they prevent access to a GP for those patients who can't afford the payment. This is less of a problem now than it was. Co-payments have fallen after a few years of focus from the previous Labour-led Government.[81] As we have already seen, historically GPs were also less likely to locate in deprived areas because residents there couldn't afford to pay their co-payments. This may well have led to a culture of less frequent visits to GPs in Maori communities.

Lack of access is a big problem. It causes the problem of 'delayed presentation': by the time the patient turns up to the doc, they are really crook, sometimes too crook for the doc to help them. As a result, we get more expensive emergency admissions later on. The rate of this kind of admissions – which are almost double for Maori and Pacific Island people – have not decreased over time. Despite the recent huge efforts made in primary care, emergency admission rates have fallen most for other races, but Maori admission rates are flat and Pacific Islander rates have even increased.[82]

It seems that access goes beyond money and having a GP nearby. Even the free parts of the health system attract fewer Maori.

The national cervical and breast cancer screening programmes are free but screening rates for Maori are 30-40% lower than the screening rates for Europeans.[83] Perhaps the most startling statistic researchers have shown is that around 35% of the difference in death rates between Europeans and Maori are due to health problems for which treatment is available.[84]

As an example of this,[85] researchers have shown that while Maori rates of heart failure are far higher, they generally receive far lower elective cardiac treatment rates than Europeans. Is this because these people have put off seeking help until too late, or because when they did seek help, they didn't pass through the system to receive treatment? This problem has been confronted and improved in Counties Manukau, as set out below.

The real question we all want to ask (but are afraid of knowing the answer) is whether our health system is racist. It's really hard to tell, but a survey of opinion showed[86] Maori have a higher reported incidence of racism within the system. While this perception by Maori in itself may impact on their health outcomes, it is not quite a smoking gun.

More recent research into treatment of heart disease[87] peels back the issues, but systemic racism is still very difficult to prove. Maori receive less treatment than others: for example they get third fewer angioplasties, half the number of stents, and they are more likely to stay in general wards rather than cardiology. Maori are 40% more likely to die on admission and the risk of death remains higher for Maori throughout their stay. This might be because they are too far gone when they arrive – adjusting the data for health problems which might complicate treatment (such as obesity), or for the rurality of the Maori population explained some of the difference in treatment, but not all. This leaves two possible explanations – there is racism present in our hospitals, or Maori get systematically lost in the health system. Both are probably partly true. Some doctors involved in the research felt the conclusion that racism was present was hard to avoid. As for getting lost in the system, we will see that our health system is not always the most organised. Sometime you need to put your hand up and shout to get care. This can be a barrier to care for those unable or unwilling to navigate the Byzantine hospital booking system. The research also indicated a dislike for travelling long distances without whanau, which may be a necessity for heart surgery. In sum, poor, rural Maori are likely to face additional barriers to receiving care – some of them cultural, some economic but the possibility that they face racialist barriers cannot be dismissed. Indisputably they don't get comparable outputs from the health system and indisputably Maori health outcomes suffer as a result.

What is absolutely certain, however, is the importance of cultural context to service delivery. Surveys indicate that Maori and Pacific Island people are more likely to use a Maori or Pacific Island health provider if the option is available.[88] Likewise, pilot studies have shown that Maori respond well to services that use Maori outreach workers.[89] It seems that the cultural context for the delivery of health services is important. This is very concerning given that numbers of Maori and Pacific Islander healthcare workers are so low, and not showing much sign of improving. In 2008, 3.2% of health workers were Maori and 1.7% were Pacific Islanders, while Maori comprise 15% of the total population and Pacific Islanders 7%.[90]

There is a lot of work to do. Improving Maori and Pacific Island health has to be a priority, not least because they are a growing proportion of our population. This should be a relatively cheap way of improving health too – prevention of disease by immunising kids and stopping smoking is far more cost-effective than giving old people hip operations. The representativeness of the healthcare workforce will need to improve also, but in the short term we will have to make up for the deficiencies by improving the cultural awareness of existing staff (particularly foreigners) and by reaching out to Maori and Pacific communities. These outreach roles will need to help guide Maori and Pacific Islanders around the healthcare system, make sure they get the care they need, and case manage patients with multiple health problems.

WHAT GE⁺S FUNDED?

If you've gleaned nothing else from this book so far, you should by now have taken away the message that publicly funded healthcare is not a limitless resource. There is not currently enough money in the kitty to fund all the treatments we'd like, all the time, and the problem is only going to get worse. That means we ration our health services. People – and for the moment, let's include politicians in this category – don't like to talk about it, but it's happening right now in a hospital near you. And it's going to be happening a whole lot more.

So once we're reconciled to this fact, we can move on to discuss the real issues. How do we decide how much to spend on healthcare and what (and whom) to fund?

Three kinds of rationing of healthcare funding currently occur. First, decisions are made as to how much money we ought to spend on healthcare (as opposed to education, roads or tax cuts); then within the health budget, decisions are made as to which treatments to fund (what you might call 'prioritisation *across* treatments'); and finally, decisions are made as to who gets treated before – or even instead of – another ('prioritisation *within* treatments').

Naturally, these discussions are not needed in private healthcare. If you want a treatment and can pay for it (either out of your pocket or through insurance), then you do. End of story. Here, and for much of the rest of the book, we're going to be talking about the public system. And we're going to leave to one side, for the time being, the question of how much money the public purse should spend on healthcare. We'll return to it in Chapter 9.

First, we're going to look at how the public health budget is divvied up. For starters, we'll look at prioritisation *across* treatments – whether we should spend the health dollar on more hip replacements or on more nose jobs. Then, we'll have a look at prioritisation *within* treatments – how we decide *who* gets the hip op, or the nose job.

What do we want from our health system?

Funnily enough, we never really ask the most fundamental question of all when it comes to the public health system. What do we want it to deliver? That's because we eschew rational debate in favour of expectation: we expect universal entitlement to every available treatment, because that's what the government has promised us. OK, so it may not be this particular government that's promised it – it was Michael Joseph Savage back in '35 – but a promise is a promise, right?

Well, it's time to wake up and smell the hospital-grade disinfectant. We're at a crossroads on this stuff, and it's time to start thinking. So let's have a look at the range of alternative options to see which one appeals.

I'm all right, Jack – A system that takes care of me and my family according to my ability to pay. I get back what I put in. This is the private insurance model, à la the United States. This is fine until you confront the issue of what to do with those who can't afford to provide for their own healthcare. In the United States, these people still receive emergency care. It's argued that this makes healthcare much more expensive, because there's no money going into the prevention of health problems. Amazingly, even though it's supposed to be every citizen's private obligation to look after their own health and that of their dependants, the US *public sector* actually spends more on healthcare per person than New Zealand does. The private sector more than doubles that spending again. And according to the measures that we have described in Chapter Three, the outputs and outcomes they get for their money are crap – ranging from absolute gold-plated services for some to absolutely nothing for others (15%, or 45 million Americans, aren't covered by medical insurance, the foundation of their health system) – hardly a ringing recommendation for this system, then!

I know my rights – A taxpayer-funded system with clearly defined healthcare entitlements. This approach is known as 'social insurance', and is similar to our ACC system. This approach is popular in many European countries. People know when they make their contributions that they are entitled to a clear set of treatments, and if they want anything else, they make private arrangements for it. Unfortunately, these systems are expensive in the first instance and vulnerable to cost blowouts when demand for treatment or the cost of treatments increase, as they have a habit of doing. We've seen it within our own ACC system recently, and doubts have even been raised about ACC's survival, given the high cost of treatments.

When the proverbial hits the fan – People pay their own way except for the really big, one-off treatments. Hospital care is free while the more preventive parts of the system – such as visits to the family doctor and dentist – attract co-payments (particularly for the wealthy). Hospitals focus on major, usually lifesaving treatments. Minor treatments that might improve quality of life or prevent future problems are ignored, or pushed into the private sector. Again, this approach tends to under-invest in prevention. This appears to be where the New Zealand system is heading.

Longer, healthier lives for all – This approach would see a fixed budget focused on activity that gave the greatest improvement in our collective health and lifespan for each dollar disbursed. Money would be spent where the biggest health benefits are, usually leading to a heavy investment in prevention and early intervention. There aren't any countries that wholeheartedly use this approach, but the UK and Canada have taken steps in this direction.

Intuitively, and given the often remarked-upon value for money that preventative health spending offers, it seems our health system should be moving in this last direction, too.

So those are the theoretical options. What do we currently do in practice?

Our unrealistic expectations mean that whenever the subject of rationing health services comes up, we're prepared to squeal like a porcupine with a needle phobia entering a hall of mirrors – and yet still apply steady, unwavering pressure on politicians to cut taxes every three years. The cake, please. And a fork.

That affects the size of health budget, as it has done year in, year out since World War II. But it also interferes in the machinery of the health system, too. While we do prioritisation *within* treatments pretty well, where informed decisions are mostly made by health professionals, our expectations make a meal of prioritisation *across* treatments. Partly this is because we have a media who are only too happy to splash stories of the casualties of rationing across their front pages, and because we have a crop of politicians who would prefer to bow to ill-informed public pressure rather than make a stand and try to explain the principles. The most glaring and potentially damaging example in recent years was John Key's ham-fisted intervention over the issue of the funding of Herceptin (see panel).

Every year, money has got tighter, and the need for change has got greater. To their credit, in the early 1990s, the National Government bravely tried to determine a core set of services that the Government would fund, in an attempt to drag us towards the 'social insurance' camp where at least you can say there's a sound basis for every rationing decision. The public would have clarity over whether to take out health insurance, and for what.

It was a nice idea, but it failed. No one could agree to dump any given treatment from the list, regardless of clear disparities in the value for money differing treatments offered. How dysfunctional is that? How craven and cowed by the dead weight of ignorant public expectations can you get? As we've seen, of all the big ideas that National tried, such as the Health Funding Authority and Pharmac, only Pharmac survives to this day.

And any progress that might have been made toward introducing a bit of reason into the debate went out the window with Labour's response, post-2000. They skilfully washed their hands of all the hard decisions regarding what to fund, devolving them – and the stain of unpopularity – onto locally elected District Health Boards (DHBs). In theory DHBs would take into account national priorities, work out what they could afford, assess local desires and needs and make sensible, pragmatic decisions as to which procedures to purchase. Yeah right.

So we're stuck with a 'system' of prioritisation across procedures that reflects the wilful ignorance of the public and the acute aversion of politicians for anything that might resemble unpopularity. Predictably, it's a mess, underpinned by emotion rather than reason.

So is there another way? Is there a rational means by which to choose where to put our scarce public health dollars?

Well, yes, there is, thanks for asking. It's called a QALY. And while you – like most politicians, as it happens – wouldn't know a QALY if it bit you and showed you its driver's licence, QALYs are out there, right now, providing a guiding star in some of the darkest, murkiest decision-making areas imaginable.

There's an important difference between the calculation that the government must make when it buys heath care and the way most commerce proceeds. When you buy something, you generally pay a price for it. You will generally only buy that thing as long as the benefit you get from it is greater than the price. Let's take beer as an example. Say the price is $5. You've been digging holes in the sun all day, and the first beer is cold, crisp and refreshing – it hits the spot. Way better than $5 worth. So you have another, and another. At some point, as you approach the bar reaching into your pocket, it occurs to you that you'd rather hang onto your $5. That, assuming beer hasn't entirely clouded your judgment, is when you stop buying it. Of course, if you've lost it by this stage, you might wake up the next morning halfway up a flagpole with a huge headache and no money in your wallet.

It's a little bit like that when the government buys healthcare. Each procedure it pays for has some benefit for society, and the government will, of course, prefer to buy procedures that offer benefits that are greater than the cost. But the whole thing is complicated, as we've just been discussing, because there's another interested party in the transaction, namely you. The government is buying the procedure for you and it could be that the procedure has a value for you that is out of line with the benefit accruing to society. This is where disappointment – and emotionally charged media campaigns – begin.

The first principle in prioritisation is that the government must ignore the value for the recipient of each procedure it funds and focus coolly on the benefits for society. With luck, the government knows the cost of each procedure (although, as we'll see later, some DHBs are so financially inept they can't even tell us that, which kind of hamstrings any sort of prioritisation discussion from the outset). But let's assume we know the cost of each procedure and that they are fairly similar across the nation. The hard part is assessing the *benefits* each procedure yields, in such a way that value-for-money comparisons can be made between different treatments. After all, if you get a patient fully back on their feet, they become a productive member of society again.

We can look at the crude cost of procedures. This doesn't allow comparison across treatments, and, even within treatments, it assumes that each procedure is of equal quality. Anyone who has been stitched up with the surgeon's watch still inside them, or had to have their ribs re-broken and reset because the first doctor was having a really bad day, knows they aren't. So we can do cost per output, such as cost per cancer screened, cost per heart attack treated, cost per appendectomy where the patient doesn't keep the surgeon's watch, etc. But the outputs of different treatments are quite different, so that here again, comparisons across treatments are impossible. So instead we could try to standardise the outputs across different treatments by working out the outcome of how much longer a treatment keeps you alive. Phew – nearly there! But even this isn't quite good enough, is it? A treatment that keeps you alive on a battery of life support apparatus and without any higher brain function can't be considered to have delivered equal benefit to the heart-valve surgery that restores you to almost complete health. We clearly need to adjust the extra years of life granted for the *quality* of that life.

The result of all this hard thinking is the QALY – or Quality Adjusted Life Year. A treatment that gives you one additional year of fully mobile life is worth 1 QALY. Conversely certain death following treatment is worth zero QALYs (so euthanasia is unlikely to rate highly on this scale). Living for part of the year, or living the full year but in a less than fully fit state is worth part of a QALY. How do we know how much people value a partial state of health? Surveys are used to determine general attitudes, and while it's only a rough and ready measure, it's better than no measure at all.

Plugging in figures for how much life a patient is expected to gain from a procedure, and adjusting for whether that life will be lived in a state of full or partial health, smart people can work out the cost per QALY of each procedure (or the amount of QALYs a certain procedure would give us for a certain cost). This is now a value that can be used to compare different treatments. So, in theory, at least, if Treatment A gives us one QALY, and Treatment B gives us 2 QALYs, and they cost the same, you'd be mad not to choose Treatment B. If Treatment A costs *exactly* half as much as Treatment B then we should value them equally. Finally if Treatment A costs *less* than half as much as Treatment B then we should choose Treatment A.

That makes all the hand-wringing and agonising a thing of the past for the government. It's simply in the business of buying as many QALYs as it can get for its dosh. And if the government is focused on this, then there's no need for any more dumb-ass and downright dangerous decisions like the Herceptin debacle.

Case study: Herceptin – a PM acting dumbly

We've all heard of Pharmac, and we know what they're there for. They're the bastards with the god complex who make flinty-hearted decisions denying young mums-of-three lifesaving chemo, aren't they?

As we've seen, Pharmac was set up in order to reduce (or at least, to limit) the rapid growth of public expenditure on drugs in the early 1990s. To do this, it goes through a process of having new drugs reviewed from clinical and value-for-money perspectives. Then it prioritises drug spending, negotiates with drug companies over price and ultimately decides which drugs will be funded with public money. And as we saw in Chapter 3, Pharmac has been very successful at constraining the growth in the drug budget.

How does Pharmac make the sort of trade-offs we have been talking about? How does it choose between a myriad of lifesaving drugs? First, it looks at the benefit a drug can generate for a person. They measure this in QALYs. Then Pharmac works out how much it would cost for each drug to generate one new QALY – to give someone the equivalent of another fully functioning year of life. This includes whether the drug reduces the cost of other health interventions, such as reducing the need for surgery.

They consider lots of other factors, too, but putting it simply, Pharmac tries to get the most QALYs within the budget limits given to them by politicians. Between 1998 and 2005, their investments on average cost around $6,800 per QALY.[91]

Pharmac doesn't give a definite dollar limit they are prepared to pay for each QALY, because they take other things into account. But as a rough rule of thumb, we can be fairly certain Pharmac would fund drugs that can give someone an extra year of full quality life for less than about $20,000, and probably wouldn't bother with anything over $40,000.

Into this logical and transparent setup barged the new drug Herceptin, with a reputation as being of some use in treating breast cancer. Backed by the wily marketing power of the drug company Roche, a highly emotional publicity campaign was mounted that managed to convince the country they were being denied access to a lifesaving medication by a conspiracy of bureaucrats and heartless politicians. The media loved it, of course, and took care not to scare up any facts that might contaminate the story. A 12-month course of Herceptin cost around $100,000 per QALY, meaning that if we were to divert precious resources into funding it, we'd be spending well in excess of the entire budget for hospital services in some of the smaller, rural areas, such as the Wairarapa and Marlborough.[92] And, of course, for every happy Herceptin customer, there were others who were missing out on quality-adjusted years of life – around five times as many – all for the want of an equally effective disinformation campaign.

For reasons that are clear only to him, John Key decided to make access to Herceptin an election issue, and Pharmac was overruled so that the drug could be funded after all. Where was his head? In one fell swoop, and before he was even in office, he'd undermined 15 years of progress and turned his back on a proven, rational approach to the thorny issue of prioritising drugs.

By hauling these decisions back into the political arena, the National Party has put the only clear and rational part of New Zealand's healthcare system back at the mercy of populist campaigns. The drug companies must be licking their lips: finally, they've found a way to crack open New Zealand's trailblazing, consumer-championing drug purchaser. They'll be laughing all the way to bank.

There's also a terrible message in this for other areas of the health system. They should shroud their funding allocation decisions under a veil of secrecy, because if they're as open and transparent as Pharmac, they'll become a target for all sorts of special interest campaigns. Better to fudge it in shades of grey.

What rationale can there possibly be for such gross, ill-advised political intervention?

The QALY is not failsafe. It might, for example, take a long time and a lot of expense to work out the QALY impact for a new treatment. Randomised trials are expensive and time-consuming. However, thinking in terms of QALYs frees prioritisation decisions from distractions. It's the approach as much as the nice detail of the procedure that is so valuable.

As it stands, all QALYs are valued equally. There's no adjustment for the relative value of an extra year of life for a young person, a mother with a small baby, an elderly person, a politician or – heaven forbid – an All Black.

This can admit some humane exceptions that might otherwise, on a strict consideration of QALYs, be excluded. A really good example of this is in the case of haemophilia. This is a rare genetic disorder – rare outside the European royal families, anyway – that prevents clotting in the blood. A simple cut or bruise can, if untreated, lead to the patient bleeding to death. The cost of keeping haemophiliacs alive usually outweighs most QALY measures that are used to justify public spending. In 2001, 69 people were treated for haemophilia at Auckland Hospital at a total cost of $5.2 million. This is about $75,000 for each lifesaving treatment, although the average cost for the 23 children within this was higher, at around $130,000.[93] Of course, it's difficult to begrudge this spending, particularly for young haemophiliacs. This is probably because it's a genetic condition, and we can all sympathise with those unlucky enough to be afflicted – we'll fund the treatment, because there but for the grace of god go we. It's also a factor that there's no alternative to the treatments currently used to keep sufferers alive.

That is to say, there is some scope for tempering decisions based on hard evidence on their effectiveness with some regard for public perception. There are ways to do this that don't hopelessly compromise the system: we'll explore these in Chapter Nine.

So much for drugs, which (some spectacular cock-ups aside)

are relatively easy to assess through clinical trials and relatively easy to cost. What about treatments in general – operations and other procedures? How do we assess these in terms of the QALYs they offer?

Effectiveness across different treatments

Given what we have seen so far, it should come as no surprise that we don't really know everything about how different healthcare interventions contribute to keeping us alive longer and in a better condition. Even when we do know something, this knowledge is not currently used to direct spending where it is needed most. When national decisions are made to increase funding and activity in a certain area, this is usually done in reaction to a specific report or scare or publicity campaign and without regard for its effect on the rest of the health sector.

We don't have space to rehearse the results of all the studies that have been undertaken on what treatments work and which don't. We'll look at a few quick highlights, then explore a few big issues in more detail. We'll finish by having a look at the thorny issue of prioritising between primary care and end-of-life treatment.

As mentioned in Chapter Three, studies in the United States and the United Kingdom suggest the two most effective (and cost-effective) health interventions of recent times have been reducing rates of smoking and providing statins (which lower cholesterol) to men with established heart disease.[94] Childhood immunisation is still a mainstay, and quietly saves the health system money. Certain carefully targeted screening campaigns can be beneficial, but this can be taken too far – prostate cancer screening is a good example[95] (despite the protestations of your League of Fathers types, who demand a national screening programme to balance the resources deployed on women for cervical and breast cancer screening). Prenatal care, drug and alcohol treatment and preventing blood-clots are also stand-outs. Interestingly, investing in medical treatment seems to be, on average, far more cost-effective than injury reduction and toxin control in improving our healthy lifespan.[96]

Big ticket items

Some work has been done in the UK for 2006/07 that suggested that the cost of saving a year of life across the main ailments were as follows:

- £ 5,425 for respiratory problems;
- £ 9,974 for circulation problems;
- £ 15,387 for cancer;
- £ 21,538 for gastro-intestinal problems; and
- £ 26,429 for diabetes.[97]

So, at least in the UK context, it is around five times cheaper to keep someone with respiratory problems alive another year than it is someone with diabetes. So if you were focusing narrowly on securing the best results for your money, it would therefore make sense to do more work on respiratory problems, and cut back on the diabetes treatments, focusing only on the aspects of treatment that worked the best. Unfortunately, no such data exists for New Zealand (although an analysis of our system could be expected to yield broadly similar results), and nor are these sorts of trade-offs made when deciding how to prioritise your healthcare money – yet.

Given New Zealand's prevalence of respiratory problems, heart disease and cancer, it seems to make sense to focus on treating these. As for diabetes, the focus should be on prevention, although for the growing number of sufferers we already have, there's emerging evidence that bariatric surgery (better known as 'stomach stapling') may be a powerful and cost-effective treatment for the obesity that underlies type-two diabetes.

Sweating the small stuff

So things look good on the main life-threatening treatments. Unfortunately they don't look so hot down at the other end of the scale. The message we got from most major hospitals is that many basic surgical treatments – including cataracts, varicose veins, haemorrhoids, hernias and mole removal – are heavily over-subscribed or simply not available in the public system. These conditions are all relatively low-cost to treat and not immediately life-threatening. However, they all bring some discomfort into the lives of those afflicted, and if untreated, they can lead to far more complicated, serious conditions. Because they are minor, they don't make big headlines if untreated. Because they are relatively cheap and non-urgent, the middle class can save up and go to private sector providers. But there is still unmet need (as the box below shows), and if left untreated these unmet needs can add up to a big health problem.

Canterbury charity hospital

Kathy is one of many volunteers who give their precious time to Canterbury Charity Hospital. Initially she did it because she had time, but it amazed her what a difference the hospital made to people's quality of life by offering simple procedures that the public sector will no longer fund. One patient was elated when Kathy called to inform him that he had been scheduled for a cataract operation. It turned out he had a fall recently and still had stitches in his head, and a cataract operation would allow him to retain his independence longer. Other grateful patients have been able to return to work following a hernia operation.

Philip & Susan Bagshaw, Randall Allardyce and Brian Stokes established the Canterbury Charity Hospital Trust in 2004 on the basis that no government would be able to meet everyone's healthcare needs. The hospital employs two staff, and everyone else is a volunteer – including doctors, nurses and technologists, as well as others in the community who help with the day-to-day running of the hospital right down to the cleaning.

Lorraine Proffit manages the hospital. She says that over and above the free service, customers appreciate the homely atmosphere and personal touches that a small hospital like this provides, complete with cups of tea while they wait to be seen. Patients even get a call the night before just to make sure they turn up – after all no-one wants to waste volunteers' time.

In its first full year of operation the hospital had consultations with 483 patients, and undertook operations on 229 people. The Trust delivered $360,000 worth of clinical services to patients in the first 6 months of this year. The existence of the Charity Hospital indicates that there is a large unmet need in the community, particularly for minor procedures amongst those who don't have insurance or the means to go private.

Sometimes the patients aren't the only ones to benefit. Such is the variety of experience provided by the collegial atmosphere at the Charity Hospital, Kathy has been able to gain skills in whole new areas of nursing, and now she has a new job as a result.

Auckland is just in the throes of establishing a similar charity hospital to that in Christchurch.

Are we missing a trick by not sweating the small stuff before it turns into big stuff? Should we fund more cataract operations to prevent the elderly falling in their homes? Should we cut out more moles to prevent melanomas? Should haemorrhoids get nipped out before they can cause clots and pulmonary embolism, even strokes? Without proper prioritisation, it's difficult to tell, but as Grandma used to say, take care of the moles and the melanomas take care of themselves.

Prevention is better than cure

We all know the old adage – prevention is better than cure. But is it? And if it is, should we do more of it? New Zealand is already a comparatively big spender on prevention and public health, as the chart below illustrates:

Figure 15 **Total expenditure on public health and prevention**

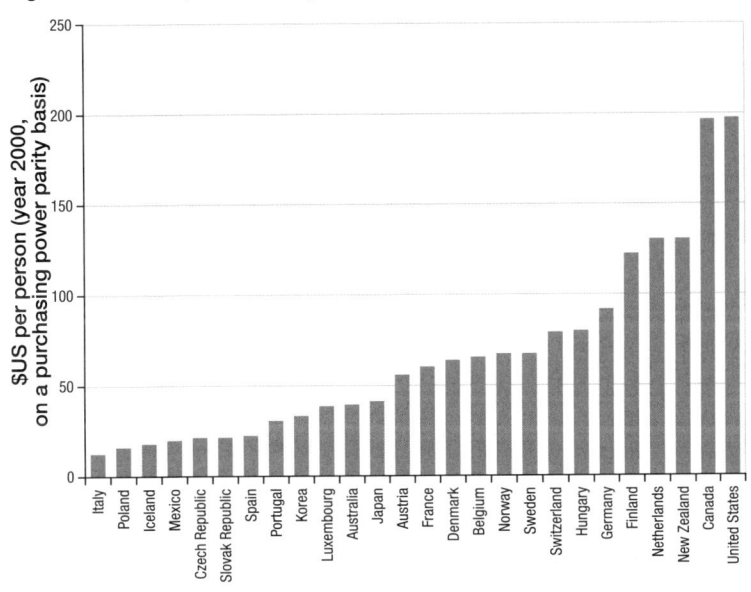

Source   OECD Health Data 2008

Given it can be very difficult to evaluate the effectiveness of preventative or public health interventions, it's politically easy to divert money away from prevention, especially when there are high-profile cases in the press of people who are dying for lack of treatment. Yet despite all the column inches devoted to the waiting lists for elective care, international evidence suggests that the real health benefits come from having a comprehensive and easy-to-access primary care system. A review of hundreds of different treatments found that preventive and primary care interventions were four times more cost-effective than procedures in the rest of the health system.[98] Yep, you heard right – *four times* better value for money! US evidence also shows there are high returns from boosting the numbers of GPs and doing check-ups to pick up diseases earlier.[99] [100] Other literature surveys have concluded that:

... primary care improves health by showing, first, that health is better in areas with more primary care physicians; second, that people who receive care from primary care physicians are healthier; and, third, that the characteristics of primary care are associated with better health.[101]

So we've got it right when our health system spends more on prevention than most other countries, although we could do a lot more still.

Dr Edric Baker

Dr Edric Baker is a Kiwi doctor who served as a medic in Vietnam during the conflict. There, he had the experience of working with locals in remote villages and was amazed at how well they coped in running their own care despite the total lack of modern facilities and resources. This awakened his vision of *health services for the poor, by the poor.* From the 1980s, Edric has devoted his life to building up a hospital in Bangladesh from scratch, training the locals in literacy and numeracy, then the basics of medical care. In 2007, they treated over 25,000 patients on a budget of $US110,000, some of which, we're proud to say, comes from the Morgan Family Charitable Foundation.

This tale of a Kiwi hero really shows what a difference simple primary healthcare can make for a relatively small investment. One of their most important programmes works with over 200 new mothers from 14 villages each year, and tracks each child up to the age of four. Their efforts are made all the more powerful when there is a commitment to getting people to be responsible for their own care – for example Edric's TB eradication programme is entirely run by former TB patients. It should be no surprise that these sorts of treatments figure highly in the cost-effectiveness rankings. In 2000, the World Health Organisation produced a list of the most cost-effective medical treatments.[102] They are almost all part of primary care or public health:

- preventing and treating tuberculosis;
- family planning;
- assistance for mothers before and during childbirth;
- AIDs prevention;
- immunisation;
- tobacco control;
- treatment of STDs, malaria and childhood diseases; and health education and nutrition.

Basic public health and primary care is by far the most cost-effective way to improve life expectancy. This may seem obvious to you and me, but it is worth reminding ourselves that a large proportion of the world's population don't even have this level of cost-effective care.

We fund all of these treatments already in New Zealand, although as we saw with Maori immunisation rates we could do more. True citizens of the world would probably worry less about getting a new hip so they can enjoy their yachting during retirement, and more about making sure mothers and children didn't die during childbirth in the Third World. We could easily lift the average life expectancy of the world if we closed a few hospitals in New Zealand and helped deliver basic treatment overseas. In New Zealand, around five babies die in their first year of life per 1000 live births, on average. This is a tragedy. The UN estimates that the average across the whole world is around ten times higher – 50 per 1000 live births. This is a travesty.

If you have a good GP, they're likely to help you prevent developing an illness, or at least spot it early. Having a good, cheap-to-access primary system ensures most conditions get picked up early, and patients don't go on instead to pop up later as expensive emergency cases. By this stage, treatment is very expensive and it's often too late to do much good for the patient. Obviously, the cheaper access is, the more people – particularly poor people – will use primary care. Greater coverage means that more people get treated, and the population is generally healthier. Contrast this with the US model, where at any given moment in time, some 45 million people have no insurance. Those with insurance get the most expensive care in the world (which isn't necessarily the best – see below) while the uninsured get nothing. The benefit (in length or quality of life) for each additional dollar spent on the rich and insured is pretty small, whereas the benefit from offering an uninsured person primary care would be immense.

There are some other reasons for favouring primary care.

Specialists are pretty good at treating conditions that fall within their hitting zone, but many people have more than one condition at a time. A specialist may well overlook something that is not familiar to them, or even exaggerate the significance of something that is (a tendency that shades into the 'supplier-induced demand' we will discuss in the next chapter). GPs, by contrast, are more likely to take a holistic approach to your care and treatment, and as the gatekeepers to the health system, they may even save you from yourself when you show up waving a printout from www.hypochondria.com and demanding treatment that is, from an expert perspective, unnecessary. A good GP or practice nurse can hold our hand and talk us down from our fear of the radiation from our microwave, or our fixation with the symptoms of whatever disease we've convinced ourselves we're afflicted by.

You may think the US model – where patients are passed from one specialist to another and subjected to a barrage of tests – is superior, in that it's better to be 100% safe than sorry. But American outcomes don't support this. It turns out that 95% certainty is an acceptable trade-off, given that we avoid all manner of unnecessary tests and procedures at the hands of overenthusiastic specialists. This actually helps our health because, surprising as it may seem, medical treatments carry a medical risk too. Medical treatments themselves are the third biggest killer in the United States, behind heart disease and cancer.[103]

Who guards the guardians?[104]

A group of US doctors were given the following scenario. A forty-year-old woman presents with chest pain after a fight with her husband. A check of her heart rate shows it is normal. The chest pain goes away. She has no family history of heart disease.

The doctors were asked what they would have done fifteen years ago, and what they would do now?

Fifteen years ago, they would have sent her home. Maybe she would get a stress test (they would measure her heart rate during light exercise, for example, like walking on a treadmill) to confirm that there's no issue, but even that would probably have been regarded as overkill. But today, the cardiologist said, she would get a stress test, an echocardiogram, a mobile heart rate monitor, and maybe even a cardiac catheterisation (sticking a tube up a vein or artery to test blood flow around the heart). The last carries a risk of death. No wonder healthcare costs have ballooned over the years.

Prevention, then, *is* better than cure, and the effectiveness of spending in the areas of public health and primary care proves it. It's a big thumbs-up to the fifth Labour-led Government, too, which in the early 2000s channelled huge amounts of money into primary care. Their aim was to get primary care – GPs, nurses, physios, pharmacists – working together with their local community in a much more preemptive capacity. Prior to their reforms, GPs were paid for each patient visit, so the sicker a person was, the more the GP saw them and the more money they made. There wasn't much of an incentive to get patients to take care of themselves. Labour changed the system so that the payment to PHOs (who operate on behalf of GPs) was based on each patient they have *enrolled*, rather than per consultation. The idea was that this would shift the focus to prevention. Labour also increased the funding significantly in order to reduce the co-payment made by patients, in an effort to improve access. As shown in Figure 16, the average levels of fees have stayed roughly stable since 2000, which amounts to a fall in real terms.

Labour rolled out its increased funding to certain age ranges and groups over several years, and it only extended to cover the whole population in 2007, so the full effects have not yet been evaluated. But on the basis of their earlier increases, the funding led to lower fees and greater use of primary care (particularly for

Figure 16 **GP consultation fees met by patient**

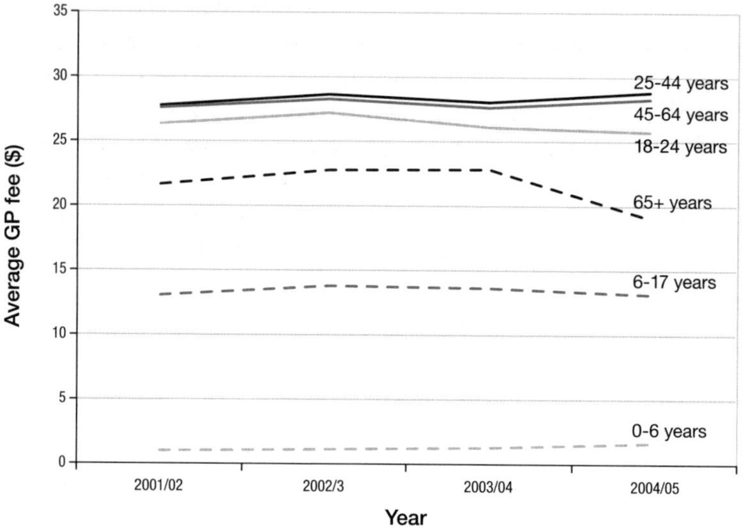

Source   Cumming and Gribben (2007)

the elderly), though not, it seems, by as much as the additional funding.[105] Their initial target areas were poor neighbourhoods, especially with high Maori and Pacific Island populations. In these areas, Labour achieved their goal of reducing fees to zero for children, $7-10 for ages 6-17 and $15-20 for adults. But in other, more affluent areas, they were seeking fee reductions for those aged 65 and over (without a Community Services Card) of $26, and average fees only fell by a paltry $12. These initial signs are worrying – over half of the new funding in affluent areas seems to have gone straight into the GPs' back pocket. There's some potential benefit – after all, we need to attract new GPs to the sector – but if affordable care can be delivered in poor areas, you have to wonder why it's not being delivered in richer areas, too. We will shortly explore how many GP practices in affluent areas may be operating inefficiently, and how Labour's cash injection may simply be prolonging their demise.

Other, early signs of the impact of Labour's reforms give rise to cautious optimism, but not much more than that. On average, people are seeing their GP more, particularly the over-65 year olds, who as a group visit the doctor 25% more than they used to – after all, it's now cheaper than calling an 0900 clairvoyant number for a chat. The extra cash has significantly reduced the proportion of people who can't access a GP because of cost – this has fallen from 4% (in 1996/7) to 0.8% (in 2006/7) for children and from 6.3% to 1.8% for adults.[106] However, the ultimate measure for improved prevention is a reduction in preventable emergency admissions to hospital, and these haven't yet shown a significant, sustained fall. Have the reforms encouraged primary care providers to practise preventive medicine, as it was hoped they would? In fact, there's reason to believe they have not, as we'll shortly see. Labour's dream was to realise Mickey Savage's vision of universal free (or low-cost) GP care. With many GPs taking a cut from any funding increases, this now seems an increasingly unaffordable goal.

How far do we go down the road of preventive medicine? There's considerable and mounting evidence, for example, that early childhood experiences (such as developing a loving bond with a mother) can have a positive impact on a lifetime's worth of health outcomes, as well as other positive stuff such, as reduced crime.[107] Evidence suggests that help to improve the mother-infant relationship targeted at young mums in high-risk communities can have a social payback of $6 for every $1 invested. Other successful programmes have used pre-school education to reach parents and children.[108] Such investments are difficult to evaluate, and at any rate, it takes many years before the benefits are known.

This kind of preventive medicine shades into the realm of social care. Health and well-being has been shown to be correlated with indicators from many other areas of life, especially education, housing and employment. Counties Manukau DHB has piloted a programme that helps mental health patients deal with these and other issues. This pilot led to a dramatic reduction in inpatient admissions, and proved a cost-effective investment overall.[109] But is this really the responsibility of the health service, or is it picking up the pieces for other failing public sector agencies? Does it indicate that it's unhelpful to have the agencies that extend help to people in need – whether it be medical or social – working in silos? Do we need to develop a more holistic approach to the whole gamut of state-provided assistance?

All this talk of the value of preventative medicine obscures another important point. Increasing investment in prevention or primary care – as the Labour-led Government did in the 2000s – is unlikely to reduce the burden of elective surgery needs on the health system.[110] This may come as a surprise – that the barrier at the top of the cliff doesn't reduce the need for the ambulance at the bottom – but it stands to reason if you think about it. The fact of the matter is that we're all going to fall off the cliff at some stage. All primary and preventive care does is *extend* our healthy lifespan, delaying the inevitable, as it were.[111] If we're putting our money into preventive and primary healthcare, does this mean we ought to be grateful for the increase in our healthy lifespan, even as we accept that resources have been diverted away from the system that will address our needs when that healthy lifespan nears its end? It probably does, but that's almost certainly not the way it will work. We'll grab with both hands the extended, healthy lifespan all that investment in primary care and prevention offers, and then bitch like crazy about the lack of resourcing of elective surgery when we reach the point when we're relying on it. And in the absence of informed debate on the subject, the government will (on past form) rush to oil the squeaky wheel.

That brings us back to the question with which we opened this chapter. Do we want a health system that maximises our healthy lifespan on the basis of need and ability to benefit (regardless of the ability to pay)? Or do we want to make sure our parents get gold-plated service on the way out? Based on the assumption that a year of life of each citizen is of equivalent value (and so the lives of the young are generally worth more than the lives of the elderly), then in terms of the value per dollar, it's a no-brainer. But clearly the good folks of Remuera and Roseneath don't quite see it that way as they face the final curtain.

End-of-life and beginning of life

Which brings us neatly to the other crucial issue: how intensively do we resource end-of-life treatment and care?

The great thing about modern medicine is that it keeps people alive longer. The bad thing about modern medicine is that it sometimes keeps people alive longer than it should. This section will focus on end-of-life, although the principles apply just as much to the beginning of life as they do to the end. Advances in medicine are constantly pushing back that age at which premature babies can be kept alive. Many of these survive to become independently viable, but unless this issue is carefully managed, some can be burdened with significant health problems throughout their life.

Overseas studies seem to suggest that, on average, a person will receive around a quarter of all the money spent on their healthcare in the last two years of their life.[112] For New Zealand, Treasury estimates that around NZ $10,000 of public money is spent on each (non-disabled) person in the last year of their life.[113] Obviously, the statistics have the benefit of hindsight – no one knows that this is the last year of the patient's life when the treatment is being extended and the money spent. Generally, though, New Zealand seems to do pretty well at capping the resourcing of end-of-life healthcare: in the United States in 1976, around one half of a person's entire lifetime health expenditure was spent in the last sixty days of their life. In 1995, studies estimated some $20 billion was spent on potentially ineffective treatment within the United States – last-ditch attempts to keep people alive, no matter the expense or the prognosis.[114]

There are guidelines and rationing procedures for some treatments, but the one glaring and inequitable exception is emergency treatment. According to Stephen Streat, who works in an Auckland intensive care unit: *'there are no national guidelines for rationing specific treatments in patients who have been admitted as an emergency (most patients in Auckland City Hospital) or who have been electively admitted and then develop serious complications.'*[115] The risk is that without careful stewardship from medical staff, patients in emergency situations could end up having the kitchen sink thrown at them.

Hasta la vista, General Franco[116]

The medical heroics performed to keep someone alive are often most apparent with the death of famous people. The vivid account of the Spanish dictator General Franco's last days is apparently fairly representative of these efforts. This is the United Press Agency bulletin of Franco's final illness in 1975:

At least four mechanical devices are being used in the battle for General Franco's survival. A defibrillator attached to his chest shocks his heart back to normal when it slows or fades; a pump like device helps push his blood through his body when it weakens; a respirator helps him breathe and a kidney machine cleans his blood. At various times in his 25 day crisis General Franco has had tubes down his windpipe to provide air, down his nose to provide nourishment, in his abdomen to drain accumulated fluids, and in his digestive tract to relieve gastric pressure... he has had three major heart attacks... undergone emergency surgery twice, once to patch a ruptured artery to save him from bleeding to death, the second time to remove most of an ulcerated and bleeding stomach for the same reason. He has taken four gallons of blood transfusion. His lungs are congested... his kidneys are giving out and his liver is weak. Paralysis periodically affects

> *his intestines… he suffers occasional rectal bleeding. Blood clots have formed and spread in his left thigh. Mucus accumulates uncontrollably in his mouth.*

We can all agree that spending a huge chunk of our health budget on people in the last year of their life doesn't make a lot of sense, and that we need to learn how to say enough is enough. But when it's Mum in the operating theatre, how can we bear to spare any expense?

It's very rarely the patients themselves who clamour for excessive and inappropriate treatment in the emergency room. The majority of patients with cancer or organ failure express a wish to die at home.[117] Generally, there's a feeling that doctors intervene more than necessary when patients want to prepare for death with dignity, and patients certainly don't want to be kept alive on life support or with less than their full mental faculties.[118] [119]

The relatives of the critically ill or injured can be a different story. The United States and Australia report a steady increase in litigation over the withdrawal of treatment at the end of life,[120] and as a result, doctors feel under increasing pressure to perform heroics to keep patients alive in all but the most hopeless of cases. As a default setting, families are fixated on keeping their loved one alive at all costs. Only a compassionate and honest discussion with medical staff informing them of the full range of choices, *including the downsides*, can help everyone arrive at the best decision. Unfortunately, not all doctors are capable of broaching such difficult discussions, and some see their role as erring on the side of continuing treatment regardless of theside-effects. People can be helped in making such difficult decisions by providing explicit guidelines from higher up in the public health system ruling out treatments that have been proven to be ineffective or too costly for too little gain in the given circumstances. It seems to be time for a 'social contract' on end-of-life treatment that would more effectively meet patient needs for a dignified death, and would probably reduce long-term healthcare costs, too.

There are many complex issues surrounding end-of-life care, and the decision to withdraw or withhold treatment. Our health system does not make it easy for people with critical conditions to set out their wishes – most of us frame a will to take care of our affairs after our death, but how many of us draw up an 'advance directive' to guide our families and our doctors in deciding to treat or not to treat when we find ourselves in limbo between life and death? And even when our expectations are set, they are too often overlooked or overruled in the heat of the moment by doctors or families desperate to hold on to a patient who is ready to pass on. This is partly a result of poor communication, culture and the design of our health system.

Doctors are trained to treat medical problems, and the public are trained to expect this. With this shared mindset, withholding or withdrawing treatment hardly seems an option. And simply caring for patients as they decline is seen by many as outside the ambit of the official acute medical system; it's the work of hospices rather than hospitals. But doctors and families need to understand that death cannot be prolonged indefinitely, and at any cost. Instead, patients need to be engaged earlier in a discussion about the appropriate balance between care and treatment.

There are three recognised trajectories you can take that end up in a hole in the ground and that put you in need of end-of-life care en route. You can be blessed with a short period of evident decline (as often happens with rapidly progressing cancer), you can suffer long-term limitations with intermittent serious episodes (as with, for example, heart and lung failure), or you can suffer prolonged dwindling (as in frailty and dementia).[121] Of course, the fourth main trajectory, which doesn't involve the palliative care specialists, is simply keeling over from some random event.

Healthy and happy one day, embolism the next. Sheesh. Yet our health system has only one approach to dealing with a terminal condition: specialist palliative care which is designed to deal with conditions where there is a short period of evident decline, and only when treatment is withdrawn. Those who work in the area feel treatment and care need to overlap, recognising a broader, more holistic and flexible definition of 'end-of-life *care*'. Evidence suggests that investing more in end-of-life *care* could even save money by reducing end-of-life *treatment*. Nurses tend to have closer relationships with the patients: perhaps part of a revamped end-of-life service would see nurses educated and empowered to assume a greater role.

Preparing for the end: a how-to guide

End-of-life situations are incredibly diverse, so it is very hard to prepare for all eventualities in advance. Yet prepare we must.

Advance directives, or 'Living Wills' set out limits on treatment in advance. These are a useful tool, but it is a question of timing. When someone is healthy, it is difficult to set out instructions which cover all possible ways of dying. Relatives can be left trying to interpret instructions in unforeseen circumstances. Besides, when The End still feels like a long way away, most of us would say 'I want every treatment known to humankind – no matter what the cost or how long the odds are'. Thankfully, the New Zealand health system is not legally bound by such flights of fancy.

As discussed above, two thirds of people experience one of three common patterns of decline and death. These three scenarios can provide a useful background for a conversation with your family on your preferences for both organ donation and end-of-life treatment/care. Such conversations are difficult, yet they are far more powerful than simple written instructions which can be open to interpretation. Once it becomes apparent that a certain manner of death is more likely, it becomes easier to plan ahead so you can give more detailed instructions. As examples, a power of attorney can be granted in dementia cases; do not resuscitate orders can be put in place for organ failure; and cancer patients can decide the most appropriate setting to receive palliative care.

Here are some top tips for end-of-life conversations:

- Get clear on what you value in life. There are outcomes worse than death, so under what circumstances would you not want to be resuscitated? If you couldn't move by yourself? If you couldn't communicate? If you lost your ability to do the 'diabolical' rated Sudoku?

- Involve everyone in the conversation, especially your kids. Your loved ones shouldn't hear about your choices when it is too late.

- Circumstances of death vary, so be wary of absolutes.

- If your doctor or nurses don't raise the topic, you should.

- Ask about theside-effects of treatment – and don't believe anyone who tells you there aren't any.

- Ask about the care options that exist as well as treatment.

It doubtless seems distasteful to many readers to be talking about money in the same breath as end-of-life treatment. But confronting the issue of end-of-life treatment is crucial to maintaining an affordable health system in the coming years and in securing a far higher benefit per dollar spent from the existing health spend. Yet it will take a sustained cultural change for families to sit down and have a mature conversation about their expectations for treatment and care. After all, most find it hard enough to discuss retirement planning and accommodation! It will also require huge changes within the health system. And above all, the public need to be more aware of the kinds of decisions that are made in the whispered, tearful conversations that take place every hour of every day between relatives and doctors at the bedside of dying patients. The media can help here: not every decision to withdraw or withhold treatment is evidence of scandalous, callous penny-pinching by health authorities.

Bravely facing the end

One health expert we interviewed for this project had a personal story that illustrates some of the difficult issues that arise in end-of-life care. Her husband developed multiple sclerosis while in his 30s. After the initial shock, the illness had the effect, as these things can do, of making everyone understand what was important in life. It gave both of them and their children the task of making a good life in difficult circumstances, a task that they faced until the end. Even so, despite their determination, his decline in the latter stages of the disease distressed him greatly. It also distressed his loved ones, as well as placing the enormously onerous burden of caring for him on their shoulders, a burden which they bore for many years. Eventually it became too much, and he was admitted to a geriatric home. This, too, was a difficult move, and he began saying he didn't want to be treated the next time he got complications. This request wasn't managed when emergencies arose, however – either medical staff forgot about the request in the heat of the moment or new staff weren't informed of it when they became involved.

Over time, his memory faded, and though his condition didn't improve, he no longer tried to refuse the increasingly invasive procedures that kept him alive. In this phase, his family were more distressed by his decline than he was – though obviously bored by his bedridden existence, his eyes lit up whenever he received a visitor. As the complications escalated, the doctors recommended a gastrostomy tube, a procedure that allows nourishment to be fed directly into the stomach. To his wife, the health expert, who was watching her husband slowly decline and sustained by increasingly invasive and humiliating procedures and with ever fewer visitors, the prospect of this continuing interminably had become unbearable. Her husband was by now unable to refuse treatment, but she and her children summoned the courage to talk to the doctors about the gastrostomy. A collective decision was made to try other ways to keep him alive. He lived nine more months without the gastrostomy, and when the next complication arose, he bravely faced the end without going to hospital and died with his family around him.

Summary

- The rationing of public health services in New Zealand isn't merely a bad dream that recurs whenever we see a face resembling Ruth Richardson's. It's real, it's happening, and it's only going to get more visible as the cloth of our resources becomes less and less adequate to cover our bulging needs and expectations.

- Rationing decisions need to be made on rational grounds. Direct political interference into poorly defined prioritisation systems is at best inappropriate and unfair, and at worst corrupt. What's more, prioritisation decisions are vulnerable to pressure brought to bear by aggressive vested interests. An equitable and rational prioritisation system will exclude these.

- The measurement of quality-adjusted life years provides a starting point for deciding a prioritisation across treatments.

- Achieving longer and healthier lives for all requires more money to be allocated to primary and preventive care. The return is four times that benefit that accrues from the same dollar being spent in hospitals.

- We need to take an unemotional view of the amount of resources devoted to end-of-life treatment, and it could well be that a more rational and humane approach would be to treat the critically ill less and care for them more. This could help them die with dignity, and also free up resources that can be better applied elsewhere in the health system.

Chapter 5

SO WHO GETS TREA+ED?

We've had a look at the way in which the system allocates resources among and within the various treatment groups, and we've underlined the importance of having a rational, transparent basis upon which to make the hard prioritisation decisions.

Now it's time to drill down a little further, and have a look at who gets treated, and how. And as we'll see, the need for rational criteria upon which to make these decisions is, if anything, even greater when you're dealing with people with faces and names than it is when dealing with groups and statistics.

Doctors have the unenviable task of weighing up life and death situations on a daily basis. None of us wants to play god in the emergency room and decide whether to save the young girl who was in a car crash and risk losing the old fella having a stroke. Doctors are guided by the Hippocratic Oath to '*apply, for the benefit of the sick, all measures [that] are required*'[122] within the limited resources at their disposal. Even if money somehow became limitless, there are other constraints, such as staff. Thus, regardless of what the public would like to believe, and what politicians would prefer to pretend, prioritisation takes place among individual cases, too, and inevitably some are steered away from treatment.

There are a number of methods doctors use to decide who gets care and who doesn't; all of the below are being used or have been used in New Zealand.

Prices

The most obvious way of reducing demand for healthcare services is to charge people. A price will naturally reduce interest in a particular treatment. The question is: who does it scare off, and why? If a price reduces demand by discouraging those with minor conditions from accessing treatment, that's probably good. If it discourages people who need treatment but can't afford it, that isn't good, either for the patient, or for the system, if the condition will require more expensive treatment down the track.

In its pure, uncompromised form, pricing is the user-pays private sector model. Some people prefer to arrange their health cover this way. However, the public system will occasionally charge patients directly, too, as with GP visits, where the state pays a portion of the cost, and leaves a co-payment for the patient to pick up.

There are problems that can arise when treatment is free – that is, when the direct cost to you, the patient, is zero. Some 9% of admissions into emergency departments around the country are for ailments that could have been treated by GPs.[123] Why? Because GPs charge, and emergency departments don't. Similarly, when there is no charge, people don't face any sanction for not showing up. Generally hospital treatment has no price attached to it, and around 9% of patients don't show up for their appointments with specialists.[124] The lack of a charge for healthcare can also encourage over-consumption and excessive expectations of the level of care available, and other such distortions. One doctor we talked to surveyed patients on why they were still in the hospital: one said he was waiting for his car to be fixed!

But there's a downside to prices, too. Ministry of Health statistics indicate that over 100,000 people are admitted to emergency rooms each year for conditions that could have been prevented by effective community services.[125] Some of these are doubtless put off going to a GP by the cost.

The typical solution when prices appear to create access barriers for people on lower incomes is some sort of extra, targeted subsidy to those who need it. Again, this has been tried for GP visits, but problems arise in distributing these subsidies. The 1990s National Government created the Poor People's Card, er, the Community Services Card, to this end. But not everyone who was eligible got one, and plenty of people who knew their way around family trust structures and the tax system got one when they patently didn't need one. Labour tried a different approach, and targeted funding to deprived areas – mostly Labour-voting electorates, as it happens, but that was surely coincidence. This turned out to be a worse idea than the Community Services Card, in terms of ensuring that people in need got treatment.[126] Why? Lots of poor people live in quite nice areas.

Labour tried again, this time hoping to move to a universal funding model where everyone pays next to nothing to visit a GP. But this was never quite achieved, simply because it's massively expensive, even if the huge investment in primary care that resulted does seem to have dropped the cost faced by most patients in accessing primary care.[127]

Given the straits our health system finds itself in, it seems anomalous that we pay for primary healthcare but there's no part-charge for hospital care. As we've seen, a part-charge was attempted in the 1990s, but it so offended the Kiwi sense of entitlement when it comes to healthcare that something just short of a citizens' revolt ensued, and the charging regime – expensive to administer as it was – was dumped before it had really bedded down.

Queues

Another popular public sector healthcare tactic to reduce unnecessary demand is to bore people into submission. Queuing was invented by the Brits, perfected by the Soviets, and has since been a cornerstone of any socialist system. The big advantage is that it is fair. One person, one vote, one place in line.

The only trouble with queuing is that the queues never seemed to get any shorter. On the contrary, they seemed to grow, year by year. In the 1990s and early 2000s, the queues seemed (metaphorically) to stretch out the hospital doors, through the car park and around the next block. If you needed an operation, your name was inscribed on the long, long list of those waiting to get one. Alas, this approach caused many problems for successive governments, because long waiting lists make you look callous and stingy when it comes to health spending. And there's a dark side to queuing, too. If you really do need the operation, things can get worse while you are waiting in line. A survey of heart surgery in the 1990s suggested that each person had a 0.28% chance of dying for every month they spent on the waiting lists. About one in forty people died because of the wait.[128] Evidence suggests there is minimal risk from a wait of about six months,[129] but this is narrowly focused on the health outcome. Meanwhile the patient has to put life on hold while they are invalided off work and warned off a whole range of the activities. The Accident Compensation Corporation finds that the longer a person is out of work, the longer it takes them to get back into work. So queues may simply push social problems elsewhere in society.

As we've seen, Helen Clark's Labour-led government was determined to tackle the problem of waiting lists, and reduced them all to six months. A miracle? Take-up-thy-bed-and-walk stuff? No. It was really no more than an administrative conjuring trick. Labour tightened the operation eligibility rules so that each DHB was forbidden to have waiting lists for longer than six months. So the DHB assesses the need of the patients who want treatment. Then they look at how much capacity they have in the next six months and – here's the tricky bit – *they set the eligibility level for an operation at the level of need that they can treat within a six month period.* So simply needing an operation doesn't necessarily get you on the surgical waiting list. Your level of need has to be sufficient compared to everyone else to get you in the first six months of operations. If your level of need doesn't quite get you on the list, you'll get sent back to your GP for what they call 'active review', where your condition is monitored. The queue has simply been shunted from the hospital back to the GP, who often has no tools to treat the patient other than painkillers.

This cute little sleight-of-hand allowed the Labour party to proclaim the end of waiting lists to a grateful electorate. In reality, no one benefited from this change. Quite apart from those whose prospects of life-changing surgery seemed to recede, the job of doctors and surgeons across New Zealand became that much harder, as they're now obliged to explain to people that although they need an operation, they don't need it enough to be eligible. Come back when you're sicker – never mind that you'll probably need a more complex and costlier treatment by then!

Need

So that raises an obvious question: how do doctors determine your level of need? For most major conditions, there's a prioritisation tool for the job, called Clinical Priority Access Criteria (or CPAC), which 'scores' a patient in terms of their need. Getting a score above a certain number on a CPAC scale means you've been adjudged to need an operation within six months. New Zealand has been an international leader in the development of these. In the majority of cases, the CPAC tools focus solely on prioritising patients for a particular procedure – they don't allow for prioritisation across different types of treatment. So, for example, CPAC could tell us which person is most deserving of a hip operation, but not whether we should do fewer hip ops and more heart surgery.

Views on CPAC, and such evidence of the scheme's effectiveness as there is, seem to vary. An objective assessment of need can be made for certain conditions and in certain areas of speciality more easily than others. For example, joint problems are generally a lot more comparable one with another than skin problems. CPAC tools thus have a varying degree of subjectivity, which inevitably means some are more open to human manipulation than others.

The degree of subjectivity can be important. If a doctor isn't confident the system will get their patients a timely result, they may find ways to help their patient jump the queue. They game the system – doctor the numbers, if you like. They know somebody who knows somebody who can do someone a deal. Great result for the patient, of course, but it results in those with the highest need waiting longer for their operations than is desirable. If enough doctors fiddle the numbers, then the treatment threshold simply gets pushed up higher over time. Monitoring is needed to ensure the consistency of CPAC scoring across the system, and this doesn't happen everywhere at present.

CPAC in Counties Manukau

Through careful implementation of the Clinical Priority Access Criteria (or CPAC) tool, Counties Manukau have managed to reduce manipulation of surgery queues and increase take-up of surgery by Maori and Pacific Island communities.

You'll remember that Labour instructed DHBs to set the threshold for treating patients at a level where waiting lists would be six months long. Doctors are concerned that people needing care will miss out, so they use the subjectivity of the CPAC tool to help those patients they think need care get over this threshold. To prevent this manipulation, Counties Manukau DHB worked with clinical staff to agree a CPAC score that would act as a treatment threshold for each condition. Over time the DHB and doctors worked together to ensure that everyone over that threshold gets seen within six months. This has improved doctor buy-in and consistency of the CPAC process.

When a Maori or Pacific Islander scores above the treatment threshold, an effort is made to make sure that person takes up their entitlement to care. Similarly, an effort is made to deal with others who do not qualify for treatment but demand it. It seems that low take-up of surgery by Maori and Pacific Islanders is partly due to the fact that they do not actively pursue treatment. In 2005/06, elective surgery rates for Maori equalled those for European/Other for the first time,[130] and the gap for Pacific peoples has also reduced. Given Maori death rates are higher from certain conditions, we should expect some surgery rates to go even higher. However, parity is a good start.

CPAC has also been criticised for not considering benefit to the patient in the prioritisation process. There are different ways to look at this. The CPAC tool does consider the clinical benefit: in other words the patient has to benefit from the procedure in order to get it. But how much benefit do we expect, and long should that benefit last? This element of benefit seems to have faded from healthcare guidelines since it had its run in the sun at the time of the Rau Williams case in the 1990s. As we've seen in the discussion on end-of-life treatment, there need to be some agreed limitations to treatment offered to people, particularly those nearing the end of their lives. To avoid charges of discrimination, such guidelines need to be based on objective evidence, such as an estimate of the number of healthy years of life that the healthcare spending generates (our old mate the QALY). This will mostly favour the young over the elderly, but more problematically, it could also militate against the disabled and even members of ethnic minorities (such as Maori) who have a lower life expectancy. It's the view of our current Health and Disability Commissioner that where there's a sound, objective evidential basis for guidelines used in prioritisation decisions, these should be defensible against charges of discrimination.[131] These sorts of guidelines are essential if we are to establish a rational system for prioritising queues. The final way of looking at benefit would be to make moral judgements about the type of person receiving the treatment. Imagine what a minefield that is. Is an extra year of a mother's life worth more than someone without children? Is an extra year of a child's life worth more than an adult's? Is an extra year for an economically active person worth more than for someone who has never worked, or who has retired? And what if the problem is self-inflicted such as a drink-driver or smoker? Moral judgements are too tough, but CPACs should at least include some consideration of the QALY benefits of a treatment.

So that's how prioritisation works in theory in New Zealand. When you draw up a schematic of how the elective surgery booking system is supposed to function, this is how it looks:

Figure 17 **Intended operation of New Zealand's booking system for elective surgery**[132]

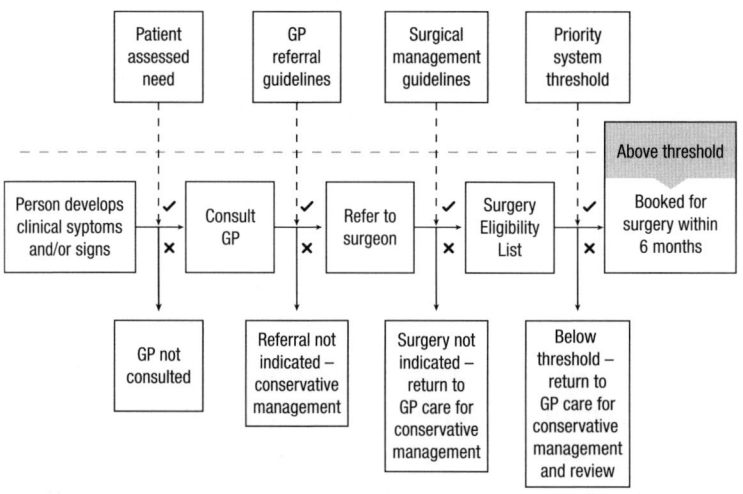

Source   Derived from Figure 6.2 in Roake J, 'Managing Waiting Lists'. In Gauld R, ed. Continuity amid chaos: health care management and delivery in New Zealand. Dunedin: University of Otago Press; 2003:107-121.

Great, isn't it? Well, yes, until you look at how it works in practice. Have a look at the graph below, which shows how long people have waited for their heart surgery and their CPAC score. In theory, if we really were applying a prioritisation according to need principle, the higher your score, the sooner you would get seen (and the closer the dot representing your operation would be to the left-hand side of the chart). But it seems the reality is very different. Indeed, according to this plot, many of the first patients to be seen are among those assessed with the lowest need. As you look at the graph, take a moment to pity the poor chap (or lady) who rated the maximum on the clinical need scale and yet took about 175 days to get an operation (her dot is indicated by the arrow). You have to admire their tenacity in lasting that long!

Figure 18 **Does treatment time reflect need?**

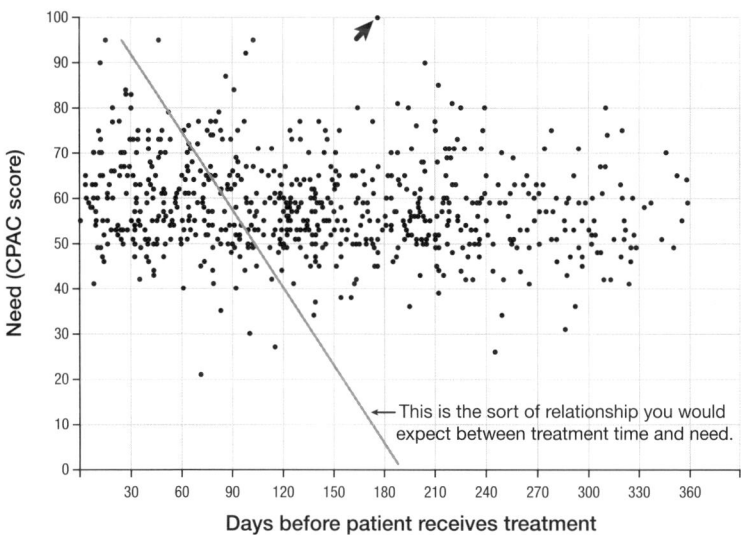

Source   Cardiac Surgery Service Development Working Group

Of course, the figure relates to cardiac surgery, and you'd have to presume that many of the patients here were operated on as the result of an emergency admission. You've been assessed as average on the CPAC scale, that is, and you're counting the days until your operation when you suddenly feel queasy and a bit short of breath. An ambulance is called, and the next thing you know, you're recuperating in a post-op ward, your surgery completed months ahead of schedule. In fact, savvy doctors make a practice of advising their patients to get admitted as an acute case in order to the jump the queue for all manner of elective surgery. Once in hospital, patients who are admitted for acute care or are occupying a hospital bed tend to get operated on first, regardless of need.[133] It's quite likely that charts depicting the timing of operations of other surgical areas would closely resemble this one. So much for prioritisation according to objectively assessed need.

The statue of Hippocrates watches over doctors today with lifeless marble eyes, but when it comes to prioritisation, the debate over how to interpret his Oath is alive and well. Some doctors are comfortable with the idea that there are limited resources, and they want to make sure they get the most health benefit for each dollar spent. These doctors will quote *primum non nocere* – first, do no harm – as a justification for erring on the side of non-treatment. The other extreme emphasises the need to '*apply, for the benefit of the sick, all measures [that] are required*'. For these docs, wherever there is life, there is hope; the mere whiff of rationing clouds this view. There is clearly a lot of work to do to get some medical staff comfortable with using prioritisation tools.

Both the Health and Disability Commissioner and the Medical Council have stated the desirability of prioritisation that's fair, systematic, consistent, evidence-based and transparent. But the example of queue jumping via acute care is one indication of how the system can be played, or dodged altogether. There are others. We'll look at each of these in turn.

Case study: Dave

In 1995 at the age of 60, Dave had a heart attack. He was in good shape, but initially thought he had bruised his rib, so in response, he upped his exercise regime to try to work through the injury. One day, exhausted and in pain, he caved in and visited the GP. She told him to hand over his car keys: he had had a heart attack and was going to Auckland Hospital straightaway.

During a heart attack, blockages in the arteries and veins around the heart prevent the heart itself from getting the oxygen and blood it needs to operate. The result is chest pain, signalling a heart attack.

Being rushed to hospital, Dave wonders what all the fuss is about. The ambulance people insist on him lying down and giving him oxygen, which he finds hilarious, and on arriving at the hospital he protests that other people in A&E must be more urgent than him. The hospital runs tests and monitors him. Within four days, he has had an angioplasty – an operation where they stick a tube in through your leg and clean out your arteries and veins. Dave greatly enjoys watching this process on the screen in the operating theatre. The doctors also put a stent in, which helps keep the artery open.

Fifteen years later, Dave is still going strong. But how urgent was his operation? Was he really an emergency or was there someone else in the community who needed the operation more? Did the GP exploit a loophole in the system to ensure Dave got timely treatment?

Another patient we talked to waited for a scan to investigate her stomach pain for over a year. She had forgotten about the scan until the pain suddenly returned, worse than before. This time her doctor tried writing "URGENT URGENT URGENT" on top of the scan request. He advised her that if this didn't work she should call an ambulance – that way she would get treatment. Turns out the triple URGENT approach worked just fine, but this ad hoc system seems a funny way of prioritising our healthcare dollar.

What gets in the way of treatment according to need?

Queue-jumping

If you manage to get an appointment to see a specialist, you could be waiting up to six months simply to find out what the problem is – specialist appointments and diagnostics can be a real bottleneck in the system. The rich and those with insurance will at this point probably opt out of the public system and go private. A handy queue-jumping alternative for the middle class is to *pay* to see a specialist who operates in both the private and public sectors. Again, a savvy GP will probably let you know about this – if you can afford to pay, that is. If you do fork out a few hundred dollars, you'll probably see the specialist more quickly, and you might even be able to get on their *public sector* operating list, so you can duck back into the publicly funded system without anyone noticing. This is one of the many opportunities to 'game the system' that result from having specialists that operate in both the public and private sector. We'll have more to say about this shortly. One patient we talked to was initially told she'd have to wait up to a year for her son's tonsillectomy – six months to see the specialist for an assessment and six months more for the actual operation. She decided to pay to see a specialist who operated in both the public and private sectors, and after the consultation, was offered the option of going on the public sector list. Then, because of a cancellation, they were able to get the operation within weeks. She has used this approach again to get her son a hernia operation.

Administration

Perversely, Ministry of Health dictates about the efficiency of hospital procedures can also have an impact on who gets treated first. Efficiency is measured by the number of different types of operations, with no adjustment for how difficult the individual operation is. In the eyes of the number crunchers in the Ministry of Health, a transplant is a transplant. But in practical terms, getting all the necessary ducks in a row for an operation – nurses, anaesthetist, doctors, equipment, theatre, post-op bed and, oh yes, the patient – can sometimes be very difficult, and the more difficult an operation is, the more resource-intensive it is. Sometimes it's just easier to do a simpler operation instead, and tick the box.

Hospital organisation is another issue. Sometimes this is out of the hospital's control – even if a patient is fully prepared for an operation and all the doctors and nurses are scrubbed and at the ready, another emergency procedure can take precedence, so that our elective patient is bumped off the list at a moment's notice –the urgent crowding out the important. This problem is increasingly being addressed with hospitals building specialist elective surgery units. But there are other cases where hospital organisation is so dysfunctional that it's administrative problems that get in the way. Referrals get lost and things change so quickly within the system that without a decent IT system, no one has up to date information on waiting times and so forth. We heard stories of patients being told that the wait for treatment would be far longer than it really was, or that they had no choice over who did the operation when in fact they did. The simple truth is that in most parts of New Zealand, people are simply not sure what healthcare they are entitled to, and how long it will take. Counties Manukau is one of the few DHBs that publicly state expected waiting times depending on a patient's level of need. Take hernia operations as an example: in some areas, hernia operations are said to be unavailable in the public system; in CMDHB, they undertake to treat all who meet their need threshold within six weeks.[134]

Geographic differences

As mentioned, the previous Labour-led Government kicked the question of healthcare prioritisation into the long grass by leaving it to locally elected District Health Boards. The Government gives most of the healthcare budget to the Boards to spend as they see fit. DHBs decide how much to spend on different activities, within Ministerial guidelines of course. Next time you're waiting for hours in A&E, make sure you use the time profitably by chastising yourself for ignoring DHB elections for all these years.

Different DHBs put different priorities on different

operations. They don't often think through what treatments offer the best health benefits. Their decisions are too often the result of history, internal politics amongst doctors, the disparate ability of personalities within the system to get their own way, and the culmination of years of the hiring and investment decisions that combine to determine hospital capacity. As a result, different areas have very different capacities to deal with different conditions. But because each DHB must only have a six-month waiting list, this means that the level of need at which each operation is offered varies wildly around the country.

There are only five centres that deal with serious cardiac procedures, for example, but where you are matters a lot. If you're in Dunedin, with historically the highest treatment rate in the country, you'll probably get the operation you need. If you're in the Waikato, with historically the lowest treatment rate, you might be better off throwing a lambskin over your back and booking an appointment with a vet.[135]

This 'postcode lottery' is contributing to a widening gap of geographic inequalities in New Zealand.[136] In part, these geographic variations are also due to the sheer numbers of DHBs in existence, and the funding formulae used to apportion money between them. We'll look at these issues in more detail in Chapter 8.

Advocacy

No system is proof against some form of manipulation, and New Zealand's health system is certainly not immune. Our interviews with doctors identified a number of sources of advocacy impacting on the prioritisation of treatment. These sources include political pressure both from Ministers' offices and DHBs, pressure group lobbying (e.g. Grey Power), special requests from GPs, media coverage and direct contact from patients themselves. Avoiding media coverage seems to be a key consideration for DHBs.

There are shades of grey around advocacy. In part, it seems unfair, because often it sees some people benefit while others – particularly Maori and Pacific Islanders, who don't speak up or don't know how to work the system – lose out. Sometimes advocacy is needed simply to get the treatment you are entitled to – either to overcome a misdiagnosis or an administrative error. One doctor we spoke to stated *'if you've still got a symptom… and are not getting an explanation that you feel comfortable with, you have to keep going, you have to keep requesting a second opinion… Most doctors these days are pleased to be challenged, they don't want to miss something…'* How many people know that?

Advocacy that helps one person may not always be at the expense of another person's treatment. Sometimes advocacy simply helps the system work better. But telling the difference between these types of advocacy in practice can be quite difficult.

Help 4 everyone?

Dorothy is a battler. She had to raise nine kids by herself after her husband died 38 years ago. As if that wasn't enough, she has lived through two bouts of cancer, one of which was in her hip. She recovered from the cancer, but her hips continued to cause her problems, which her GP treated with painkillers.

In 2008, when Dorothy was 79, her youngest daughter Jen got fed up with the constant pain she saw her mother in. She took her to a specialist and, sure enough, it was determined that Dorothy urgently needed a double hip replacement. Jen was assured that they would hear from the hospital in a week, and the case was so urgent they should get public treatment within three months. There was no need to go private.

A month later, they'd heard nothing. Jen didn't know whom to call. When she called the hospital, she was passed around to different people. No one seemed to know what was happening.

Jen knew Kay Poulsen from Help4U, a private health advisory service, and decided to give her a go. Kay swung into action, and discovered that Dorothy wasn't on any list: the paperwork had been lost. This was re-sent, and two weeks later, Dorothy had a physio assessment that confirmed the urgent need for an operation. By the end of April, still nothing had happened. Kay discovered that the fact both hips needed to be done was causing the public sector scheduling problems. Meanwhile, Dorothy's health was deteriorating. A prolonged wait might hinder her recovery. Kay struck a deal with the hospital: they would go private for one hip, as long as they could get the other one done in the public sector as soon as possible. By September both hips were done. Kay also helped to organise respite care for Dorothy to help her recover, including physio, for which Dorothy was very grateful.

Without both Jen stepping in, and Kay's help in navigating the system, Dorothy could still be waiting for her operation, despite having been assessed as in urgent need of it.

After a career in the health service, Kay Poulsen set up Help 4U to assist people in navigating its labyrinthine structures. There's a charge of $50 per query, or $200 per year for her assistance. This service has been termed by some as 'queue-jumping', but Kay's focus is on 'helping the health service work more efficiently' and deliver better results to its customers. Unfortunately, it seems that the structures of the health service are so complex that even GPs – the traditional entry point to the health system – struggle to help patients find their way around.

Names have been changed, except for Kay.

So all-in-all, continuing to focus on need seems to be the best way to decide who gets priority access to a specific treatment. CPAC is not perfect – but then, no rationing method is. Continuous improvement of the tools is all that we can ask. Meanwhile, doctors need to buy into the process and start to use the tools rather than gaming the system. A starting point could be to agree a target treatment threshold for each treatment among doctors and aim to align that with the financial threshold. This would help to reassure doctors that we are aiming to treat everyone who really needs it. Doctors may also need to work together to ensure that CPAC scoring is more consistent. Obviously, once agreed, the system needs to be audited and estimable penalties imposed on doctors trying to cheat.

The big question is how to make sure the CPAC approach actually gets used. As a starting point, the health system needs to be de-politicised, as we shall discuss later in Chapter 9. Consumers also need to be able to access the treatment they're entitled to. A decent IT system might make the health system a lot easier to navigate. An alternative is help for patients to navigate their way through. Currently, there is a Healthline phone service where you can talk to nurses 24 hours a day (on 0800 611 116) to get some initial advice on your health and where you might go for treatment. Perhaps this concept needs to be broadened into more of a Help4U-style service, where the Healthline nurses can help guide you around the maze that is the health system.

The system may sound like a bit of a mess. But we have to remind ourselves that every country in the world struggles with this stuff, and no one has the 'right' answer. New Zealand prioritises treatment pretty well – and would do better if the sensible prioritisation system we have was more widely used.

Summary

- It's just as important to apply rational, transparent principles to prioritisation decisions regarding who gets treated, too. The present system aspires to treat people according to need.
- The present rational system that we have for determining who gets treated – the CPAC score for 'need' – doesn't work, because there are too many dodges. We need to restore doctors' faith in it, and ensure everyone focuses on making it work rather than looking for ways around it.
- CPAC needs to include guidelines so that before a person receives certain treatments, the doctor is satisfied those treatments are likely to add sufficient years to someone's life to make the treatment worthwhile.

Chapter 6

PAST, PRESENT AND FUTURE – THE BIG HEAL⁺H SYSTEM TRENDS

This section looks at the big long-term trends in the health sector, with a particular focus on spending. What issues have driven the cost increases in our health system, and what will drive them in the future?

Share of our income spent on health

Health is already one of the biggest ticket items on our Government's shopping list, and has recently been growing fast – faster than many of the other items. Remember the scary graph in Chapter Three, showing how health spending had increased since 1925? Brace yourself: the news as we look ahead is even worse.

As mentioned above, recent spending increases have hit 8-10% per year. If we keep that rate of increase up, health spending would swallow half of our national income by 2050.[137] Treasury undertakes long-term projections of the government books every four years. This sort of crystal ball gazing is fraught with difficulties, but the results show the logical destination of our current path. Rather than viewing this as a 'prediction' it should simply be viewed as projecting forward current trends. It's a bit like keeping your head up when you're running: if you see you're running into trouble, you can change direction. If we don't like what the projection is indicating, then perhaps it's time we changed our heading.

According to the Treasury projections, Ministry of Health spending is expected to eat up double its current share of national income – from around 6% in 2006 the Ministry as our agent will require 12% by 2050.[138] As shown by the graph below, if *all* health spending follows that same trend (that is, including ACC and your direct, out-of-pocket expenses), by 2050 health bills could eat up a massive 18 cents out of every dollar you earn. And this is by no means the worst-case scenario. Indeed, the Treasury projection is actually conservative, and builds in some money-saving assumptions. If things really continue as they are now, they could be a lot worse by 2050 than the projection suggests.

Treasury assumes, for example, that to get away with a mere doubling of our health spending by 2050, expectations of treatment will have to fall into line with our incomes. That's a big call, given the rate at which it's rising, and our expectations (as we'll shortly discuss). Without a little recalibration of our attitudes, it's not hard to see our health bill exceeding 20 cents in every dollar this economy earns by 2050.

Some international research even indicates that healthcare expectations increase 25% faster than income.[139] If anyone has projected forward the cost of this scenario in New Zealand, they haven't passed on the results. Perhaps they're slumped over their calculator somewhere even now, still rigid with the shock.

And in case there's anyone out there prepared to argue that the runaway health budget is merely public sector spending gone mad, remember that the rises in public sector health spending we have seen in recent years have been *matched* by the private sector. So there is every reason to expect that this trend will continue, with demand for healthcare inexorably rising until… when? We get our employer to deposit our salary directly into our doctor's account?

By these numbers, health spending could easily get so big it would start to choke the whole economy through the higher taxes needed to fund it. See? That's the value of projections. While they won't necessarily happen, they show us that our current approach is unsustainable: they show us the wall into which we are running headlong.

Figure 19 **Past, present and future of healthcare spending**

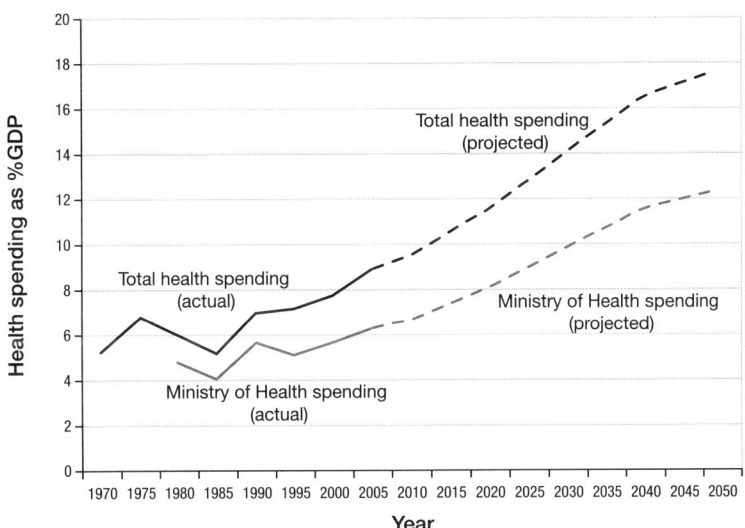

Sources Ministry of Health (2008), Treasury (2006), OECD Health Data (2008), Infometrics

The main drivers of the ballooning health spend

So what can be done? What we need to know is what is driving these cost increases. There are plenty of good reasons why we should expect the growth in health spending to continue as it has done over the past decade (or even get faster). These include an ageing population, rising expectations, new technologies becoming available, poor productivity and chronic conditions spreading through the population. We'll explore each in turn.

i. Ageing population

People in poor health, particularly those in the last year of their lives or in a permanent state of disability, tend to absorb a higher share of health spending. As people age, they are more likely to tick both these boxes, and therefore health spending generally tends to increase dramatically with age to around five times the cost of care for younger folk, as shown in the chart below. We mention in passing that the health system spends more on each woman than it does on each man – not only do women live longer, they get more healthcare spending! Let no one accuse our health system of sexism!

Figure 20 **Healthcare spending by age & gender**

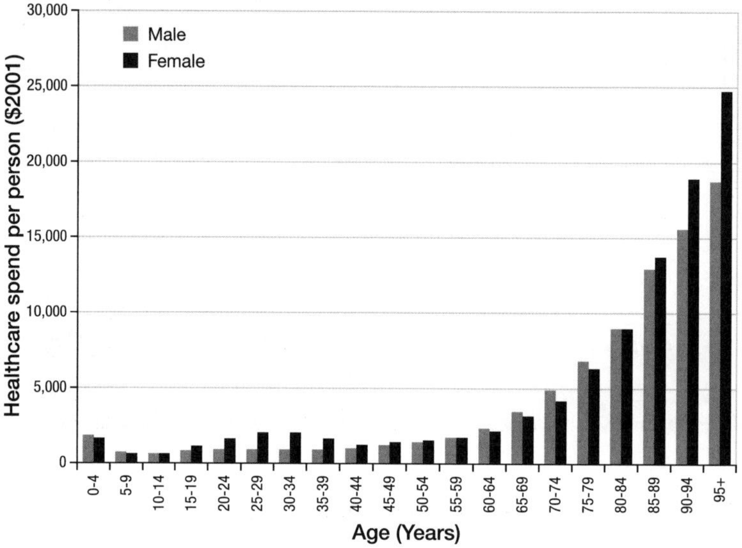

Source   Ministry of Health

As the tidal wave of ageing baby boomers hits retirement, it follows that there will be an increase in the number of people dying and living in a state of disability. Simply by having more elderly people, our health costs will start to balloon. This won't happen as quickly as the rise in the bill for New Zealand Super around 2011, but as the baby boomers hit their mid-70s (around 2020), the effects will increasingly be felt. By 2028, almost 50% of health spending will be on people aged 65 and over.[140] The share of population aged over 65 is predicted to rise from 9% in 1950 to 26% in 2050. If Ministry of Health costs do indeed double from now as a share of our income by 2050, this sort of demographic change is projected to be responsible for around one quarter of the total cost increase[141] in the health budget. Doctors' waiting rooms and hospitals will be choked by a sea of purple rinses, Zimmer frames and wrinkled faces alight with a sense of entitlement.

The graph below shows how dramatic the change will be:

Figure 21   **Geezer glut: healthcare spending by age group**

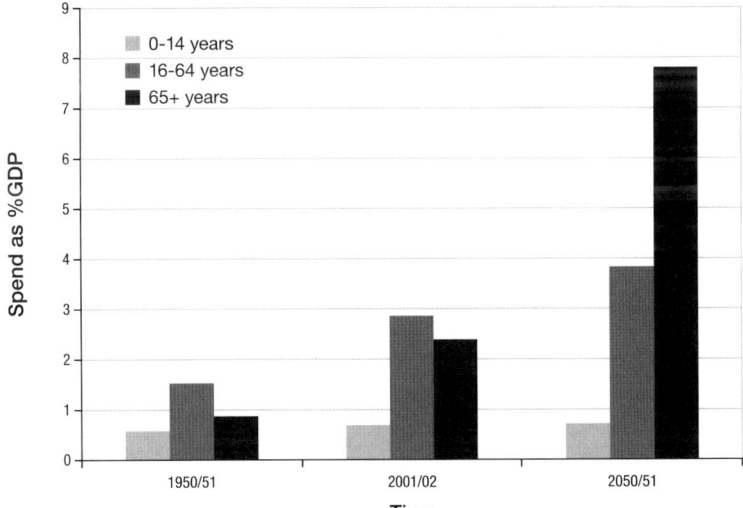

Source   Treasury (2006), Infometrics

We're fortunate indeed that this is one area where improved healthcare technology and generally higher standard of living will help. It seems we'll stay healthy for longer as our life expectancy increases, that so-called *compressed morbidity*. If this trend indeed eventuates (and that is a big IF, one that deserves capital letters), it should mean that spending on each elderly person will increase more slowly than for other age groups. This is good news: otherwise the costs of dealing with the ageing population could be huge.[142]

The moral of the story? Better be nice to your kids and hope they don't mind taking care of you, because the intergenerational battle is coming. Anyone remember the Carousel in *Logan's Run*?

Perhaps the greatest challenge likely to arise from this monumental demographic change is geographical. Some areas will face large growth in the numbers of their elderly at the same time that they're facing big population increases: Greater Auckland is worst hit in this respect, although the Bay of Plenty looks likely to suffer from it as well. Will the Jafa bashers have something to say about more resources going into Auckland to prepare for this? We'll have more to say on this later.

ii. Gimme Gimme

As we all grow richer (generally speaking) over time, our expectations, wants and needs tend to change. Maybe you've switched from instant to freshly ground coffee, or from eggs laid by battery hens to free rangers. Maybe you were happy to drive around in a banger while you were scraping together the money for a deposit for a house; now you wouldn't settle for anything less than the latest model every year.

Hordes of economists and marketers are paid to study these sorts of changing patterns of spending. Generally, as our income rises, we tend to spend a smaller proportion of our income on feeding ourselves. Meanwhile, we sink more of our money into entertaining ourselves. This sort of analysis seems to apply equally to national spending as it does in the household. For example, in 1957 British people spent 33% of their income on food, and 7.5% on recreation and culture. By 2006, the proportions had changed to 15% on food and 12% on recreation and culture.[143] Clearly, food is more important than entertainment, but once the need for food has been met, the theory goes, your priorities change and the income starts going elsewhere. That's why food gets called a 'necessity' and entertainment a 'luxury'.

You probably think that healthcare is a necessity, right? Wrong! Most international studies show that national health spending rises *at least* at the same rate as our national income.

Some indicate healthcare spending rises *faster* than income, and indeed, we've seen it doing precisely that in New Zealand. To economists, this seems odd. Once basic health needs are met, shouldn't we be happy that we're healthy and can spend our next buck on something else? In other words, wouldn't we expect to see healthcare dominate our spending when we are relatively poor (as food does), and drop away as income rises? Things just don't seem to happen this way.

To make sense of it, we turn not to researchers but to Monty Python. The movie *The Meaning of Life* shows a group of doctors (and their patient) fixating upon use of the latest technology, particularly the machine that goes 'Ping!' This story rings true – we all want the best healthcare we can afford: we wouldn't want to be picked up in a 1965-vintage ambulance, nor do we want these days to recuperate in rooms with 1960s décor (and the fact that some of us do without suffering adverse effects is beside the point). We want our healthcare to 'keep pace with the times', to take away the pain by providing our hospital beds with flat screen TVs, restaurant-level meals and nursing staff who are easy on the eye. Not a lot to ask, is it?

Demand can be driven from the other side, too. There's a well-documented phenomenon called *supplier-induced demand*, where it's been observed that doctors tend to find – and treat for – conditions that aren't really present. Why? Well, let's just say that in the United States, it's been shown that in those areas with more surgeons, more operations happen per person. And soon after a Medicare fee reduction – that is, doctors were told to lower their prices – the number of consultations went up, with the effect that 37% of the income lost through fees was recouped. There are six times more MRI scans performed in the US than here. Private sector doctors in Victoria, Australia tended to deliver more procedures to each of their heart patients, without any noticeable improvement in outcomes for the patient. It's the same situation as when you take your car to a mechanic, who frowns, strokes his chin and makes expensive 'Tsk, tsk,' noises. How are you supposed to know if you really do have problems with the camshaft's dwell angle, any more than you know if the dentist really is drilling a cavity in your tooth, or if the colonoscopy you've been ordered to submit to is really necessary?

And it's not just doctors. The pharmaceuticals industry is a past master at creating demand out of nothing. How many people would put up with theside-effects and risks that attend their blood-pressure and cholesterol-lowering medications if they were told the real risk of having a stroke? It's become common for people to present to their doctor with a list of the medications they should be on, influenced by drug company advertising. And the drug companies offer all kinds of incentives and inducements to doctors themselves for prescribing their product: it goes far beyond the branded coffee mug and the company monogrammed stationery they're using. This is just one of the reasons antibiotics are overprescribed, and often prescribed to patients who have no need of them – those suffering from viral complaints, for example, against which antibiotics are useless – risking harm to the patient and the generation of antibiotic-resistant strains of bacteria.

To cut a long story short, then, there's a whole raft of reasons why the population is subjected to unnecessary medical procedures that don't have anything to do with patient need. It's generally not such a problem in a public system, where medical staff are on salaries, but money is not the only incentive. Prestige, justifying a unit's budget or simply a love of boy's toys – doing procedures and using new technology – can all be reasons for overtreatment. So supplier-induced demand can happen in the public sector too. There's evidence, for example, that heart bypass surgery is no more effective than intensive medical treatment (i.e. all the things you can do for heart disease without cutting someone open) for people with diabetes.[144] But try telling that to a heart surgeon. This is the problem – certain treatments can become entrenched in the healthcare system regardless of their effectiveness or the availability of alternatives. Some experts also told us that surgeons often lobbied for the latest technological treatment to be made available through public healthcare simply because it was cutting edge, rather than because it was particularly effective. Aortic valve insertion surgery was cited as the latest example of such chest-thumping, alpha male surgeon antics. Some of them just can't wait to get their hands on the machine that goes 'Ping!'

It's not that we're getting lots more treatment, but the treatments we do get are far more intensive than they used to be. Looking at hospital discharge data, the numbers of high-cost discharges have been growing far faster than plain vanilla medical and surgical discharges. If we adjust for population growth, age and changes in cost weightings, the total number of hospital discharges grew by around 18% between 1991 and 2005, while high-cost discharges grew by over 50%.[145]

From the patient's side, it doesn't help that we aren't paying for the care. This allows our expectations to rise unabated. Why not consume it, if you're not paying for it? In fact, you might as well keep consuming it until you squeeze all the benefit you possibly can from it.

The lack of a price to make us think before we buy can also mean that while people have high expectations of a service, they end up valuing it less. As we have seen, some people don't turn up for their free hospital appointments. Free emergency care also encourages some people to avoid paying for a GP and go straight to hospital.

The lack of a user price for healthcare has a wider impact on our attitudes, too. As pointed out above, when the price is zero, the incentive is to over-consume the service. You keep consuming until you get no benefit from consuming any more. If we had to pay for our own healthcare, many of us would probably settle for the budget option. However, when someone else is paying, it's easy to demand the best healthcare around. We'd all drive a Lexus if someone else were paying. But if we're paying for it ourselves, most of us will settle for a nice reliable Toyota Corolla.

Surely our unrealistic expectations are the first thing that has to go if we're revamping our health system? After all, while we're demanding the earth of it, we're rubbing shoulders with people for whom a simple dose of the public health basics – decent housing, sanitation, nutrition, a job – would work wonders. We prefer, it seems, to wait until these people become an emergency before we act, and then it's to lay on expensive treatments worth many times what it would have cost to prevent. An ounce of prevention is worth a pound of cure, after all, even in today's money.

iii. The rise of the machines

The difference between man and the animals, as a philosopher once put it, in the quaintly gendered language of the day, is that man knows he's fastened to a dying animal. This gives rise to other differences between man and the animals. When did you last see an animal buying wrinkle-reducing cream, for example, or whole herds of animals spending their lives trying to develop lifesaving drugs, or the elixir of youth?

New technology can have many possible impacts on our health system. It can make an existing procedure more effective, and possibly even cheaper. But examples of technology bringing about an actual cost reduction are rare. They tend to be limited to vaccines, and other measures that prevent the need for medical attention later.

Generally, technological advances actually increase the coverage of the health system by treating previously untreatable conditions. By the time the last guinea pig has been sacrificed in the name of improving the technique, the cost per procedure has usually come right down. That must reduce costs, right? Well, not really. By this time, Joe Public has got wind of the new procedure, and is queuing up to be fitted with the latest bionic part. Volume effects then tend to outweigh the reduced costs per procedure. And the final irony is that the treated person now lives longer, and in living longer, is available for other medical care, all of which comes at a cost. Extending life expectancy through cures for conditions is a cost-raising exercise.

A spiral threatens. Where's the circuit-breaker that will save us from the treadmill of saving people from illness just so that they can go on to become ill and in need of saving? Sure, we've heard of user pays and we've seen it work in some contexts, but it's a violation of human rights in the health sector, isn't it?

Take heart – modern medicine works, but at a price

One of the best examples of how modern medicine saves lots of lives – and doesn't save money – is the treatment of heart disease.

Up until the 1960s, caring for coronary heart disease was cheap. That's because pretty much nothing could be done for the patient other than to put them in bed, drug them up to take care of the pain and hope they could ride out the storm. Usually they didn't.

Over time, this situation has changed dramatically. First, doctors could do an angiography – basically putting a little camera inside to see where the blockage is in the arteries. This opened up a whole new world of understanding about coronary problems, but it was expensive. Then heart/lung machines allowed bypass surgery. Again, these were hugely expensive but saved the lives of patients.

Then the angioplasty procedure allowed doctors to clean out fatty deposits in the arteries, producing similar results but without the need for open heart surgery. As it became more reliable, it became a cheaper procedure than open heart surgery. But the non-invasiveness of the procedure saw huge numbers of new patients who weren't willing to risk open heart surgery knocking at the surgery door. Over the same time period, a range of preventive drugs has also been discovered that help reduce the prevalence of high cholesterol and other risk factors.

Clearly these developments have dramatically increased the length and quality of life for many people. Deaths from heart disease in New Zealand have fallen by a staggering 60% since 1970. This is a remarkable achievement – good on you, health system! But what's the reward for our hard-working doctors and nurses? A whole sub-population of people who now need ongoing monitoring and medication, and usually more treatment, eventually. The health system, of course, bears the cost. It's a depressing thought, but every time such a patient is successfully checked out of hospital, it signals a larger national health bill for their ongoing maintenance and support.

It's hard to measure exactly how much technology has contributed to rises in healthcare costs, although an American study suggests it's around half.[146] The New Zealand estimates are lower, but they're still high.

iv. Baumol's cost disease

In the 1960s, a chap called William Baumol had an idea that would revolutionise the way we looked at health costs. Generally, the wages and salaries we pay ourselves rise in line with the amount of output each of us creates and sells. Baumol noticed that this wasn't necessarily the case in every industry. Wages rise in some industries, but without a rise in productivity underpinning it.

Baumol noticed that it takes the same number of musicians to play a Beethoven quartet as it did in Beethoven's time (in case you were wondering, that would be four). And it certainly didn't appear to Baumol that they are doing many more concerts than they did in Beethoven's time, either, or that any given quartet was working harder during the recital of a given piece. The wages of people playing in Beethoven quartets had certainly risen since the 18th century, however. How could this be?

He reasoned that their wages needed to keep pace with the productive sectors, otherwise everyone would want to be a farmer and no one would want to be in a quartet. So quartet musicians got paid more, even though they hadn't changed their output in 200 years. This theory then got applied to many other important parts of the economy – to any activity we as a society adjudge to be important even though those employed in it might not improve their outputs as quickly as more productive sectors. It was quickly realised that Health and Education might fit this profile: they are so important to society as a whole that rewards to providers must keep up with the wider economy if we're to attract and retain workers within them.

In reality, the theory has held rather more true for health than for education. Between 2003 and 2008, public and private sector labour costs increased by around 15%. Education sector pay rose slightly above this average, while healthcare labour costs soared by over 25%.[147] It's pretty hard to argue that these increases in health and education pay packets are in any way linked to productivity improvements.

There are two possible ramifications from the fact that incomes increase faster than productivity. We either cut production and retain fewer people in these roles over time or we (as a society) devote an increasing proportion of our national income to funding people in these roles. For quartets, we choose the former solution (there are fewer string quartets around than there used to be). But for healthcare, it seems we choose the latter.

Treasury has done some work to quantify the effect of this sort of cost increase together with the coverage increases brought about by new technology. In the past, these factors may have contributed around a third of the increase in our healthcare costs. In the future, Treasury assumes that our nation will slowly get on top of these costs, but if we don't, the long-term growth of health spending will be even higher. Ministry of Health spending alone could be 15% of our income by 2050 – this is a 150% increase on today's (6%) share, instead of the mere doubling that Treasury predicts will occur.

There's currently no sign that we'll be able to tame technology and other cost increases, as Treasury assume. In their Brief to the Incoming Minister, the Ministry of Health claimed that the public health system needs annual spending increases of around 4% simply to keep its head above water, what with inflation and population increases. With a cost structure like that, getting bang for your buck is always going to be tough.

Are we doomed to slinging more money into this black hole, or should we start to expect our doctors and nurses to get more productive?

v. Chronic health problems and 'Affluenza'
But wait! There's more!

A 'chronic' disease is one that persists for a long time. In other words, you can't just take some medicine and bed rest and get over it. Surveys indicate that just under half of New Zealanders have a chronic health condition,[148] such as diabetes, heart disease, hypertension, Alzheimer's disease or cancer. People with these conditions account for around 70% of health costs and 80% of early deaths.[149] UK evidence suggests that just under half (45%) of those with chronic conditions have more than one condition – often because one chronic condition creates another: diabetes, for example, can cause circulation or sight problems. The technical term for this tendency of diseases to hunt in packs is 'co-morbidity'.

The key growth areas of chronic conditions are amongst communities with the poorest health outcomes – so they are likely to make things worse for Maori, Pacific and low-income health outcomes. Treasury notes that *'people with chronic diseases participate less in the workforce, retire earlier, and are likely to work less productively (and die prematurely)'*. According to the National Health Committee, chronic conditions *'are the leading cause of preventable morbidity, mortality and unequal health outcomes'*.[150] The World

Economic Forum rates a blowout in chronic conditions as one of the main risks the developed world faces in the 21st century – both in terms of what they'll cost and in terms of the likelihood they'll occur.[151]

The National Health Committee and Ministry of Health provide some examples of common chronic conditions and how prevalent they are:

- chronic neck or back problems (one in four adults)
- mental illness (one in five adults)
- arthritis (one in six adults)
- heart disease (one in 10 adults)[152]
- medically diagnosed diabetes (one in 20 adults)
- asthma (one in seven children and one in nine adults).[153]

Chronic disease levels have been on the rise for some time and are going to get worse in the future. Part of this is due to the ageing effect already discussed, but part is due to unhealthy modern living – poor nutrition, smoking and lack of exercise. Between 2001 and 2011, the prevalence of diabetes is expected to rise by 60% for European New Zealanders, and over 130% for Maori and Pacific Islanders.[154] Australian projections indicate that the likely growth areas are diabetes (due to obesity) and dementia (due to the ageing population). Australian diabetes treatment is expected to rise by 436%, and dementia by 364%[155] by 2033. In New Zealand, diabetes costs are expected to triple in real terms by 2021 to $1.7 billion, although increased prevention and early detection may reduce this if investments are made now.[156] As noted in Chapter 3, the most worrying drivers behind chronic disease are obesity and our national sweet tooth.

The biggest study in recent times on the future of chronic disease was probably the UK's Wanless Report. This urged increases in public health spending to prevent the chronic disease burden impacting on future health costs. The impact is massive – they calculated that strong action by government and the public could save the taxpayer healthcare costs equivalent to 2% of national income by 2020.[157]

There are already some signs that the design of our health system (and health systems overseas) are struggling to cope with chronic conditions. Chronic conditions demand holistic care, but they often straddle many medical specialities, making coordination very important. Unfortunately, only just over half of those with a chronic condition have a plan to help them self-manage their condition, and many don't receive the necessary regular checks. Only a third of doctor's offices have a nurse involved in the care management of patients with chronic conditions, and only one third of patients receive counselling on diet and exercise. There's enormous scope for coordination problems – fewer than half of doctors take an overview of the medication given to a patient by various specialists. The cliché of an elderly person taking two suitcases on holiday – one for her petticoats and one for her pills – is not always an exaggeration. It's in fact quite possible that no one really knows about all the pills she is taking. Generally speaking, most countries have failed to cater to the multiple needs of chronic patients by bringing various specialities together into a single package of care. Only the UK seems to have made any headway toward this particular goal.[158]

Despite the rise in diseases like diabetes, no increase in the prevalence or the rising cost of dealing with chronic conditions has been built into current Treasury costing models. They are expected to be offset by lower smoking rates and falls in other conditions, such as heart disease, meaning the overall impact from increased disease rates is predicted to be small. As set out above, the key driver of cost really is the increased treatment we expect for each condition we get. The impact of obesity on our health services is the real wild card in all predictions for the future.

Summary

So overall, there are many good reasons to expect healthcare spending to continue to rise at the same rate it has in the past, and faster than our income growth:

- The ageing population
- Technology changes
- Salaries rising faster than health sector improvements
- Increasing expectations (as incomes rise)
- Chronic health problems and unhealthy modern living, especially the 'obesity epidemic'.

Surprisingly, the crucial issue isn't our ageing population as you've probably been led to believe. It's our rising expectations. Most of us labour under a delusion now if we think that our system can afford anything we want in the way of medical treatment, no procedure too tricky or expensive. To imagine that it will keep pace of our expectations in the future is just plain nuts.

There will be more old fogies in years to come, but they will be generally fitter and we are, after all, getting better at looking after them. But both the old fogies and the youngsters alike expect to be treated – more and more – for conditions that we never used to treat. And as we saw in Chapter Three, this extra treatment provides only marginal benefits, so we all get disappointed. What is it about us that prompts us, when we're confronted by this failure, to demand more rather than to stop the bleeding?

Is there no way to cut our losses? And if not, is there a way we can ensure we start to see the benefits of all this extra money going into the health system?

Chapter 7

LET'S PLAY DOCTORS AND NURSES – THE HEAL⁺H SECTOR WORKFORCE

All the advances in the drugs and technology of modern medicine haven't changed one essential truth: it is the people – the health sector workforce – who determine whether your system works. Without competent doctors and nurses, all the drugs and machines, all the bricks and mortar, all the systems and administrative excellence in the world will avail us nothing.

It's got to be a worry, then, that the health experts interviewed for this project commonly identified workforce issues as the biggest facing the sector.

Past governments abrogated responsibility for health workforce planning, figuring that the market will provide. Once it became apparent that there was no invisible hand on the tiller (and no fairies at the bottom of the garden), the Medical Training Board was set up to do some actual steering.

This chapter will look at the workforce issues facing the health sector, both perceptions and the reality. Do we have a 'shortage' of doctors and nurses, and if so, which areas feel them most acutely? Are doctors really obstructing the recruitment of staff overseas to keep supply short and prices high? Are we really training medical staff just so they can jump ship and take up more lucrative positions overseas? Have student loans made the problem worse? And what about all the foreigners we see wearing white coats in our hospital wards? Do they really know what they're doing, or are we getting what we pay for – second-rate medical and nursing staff who can't get proper jobs elsewhere? Am I safe entrusting myself to their care?

Supply of health workers

Comparing the health workforce in different countries is notoriously difficult, because different health systems work in such different ways. Responsibilities between doctors and nurses vary, and even the way the system functions differs. In the US, for example, there are very few GPs and lots of specialists, whereas here and in Britain, we have a large network of GPs who act as 'gatekeepers', controlling our access to more specialised care. We've already noted elsewhere that like most other Anglo countries, we have comparatively more nurses and fewer doctors. It can be hard to say what is the 'ideal' number of doctors, nurses and specialists the system should have.

Despite the headlines about staff shortages in the health sector, the numbers of every kind of medical worker (apart from pharmacists) have been growing steadily – faster, in fact, than the general population, and for as far back as records go. This is how the numbers of nurses and doctors look over time:

Figure 22 **Practising nurse and doctor workforce**

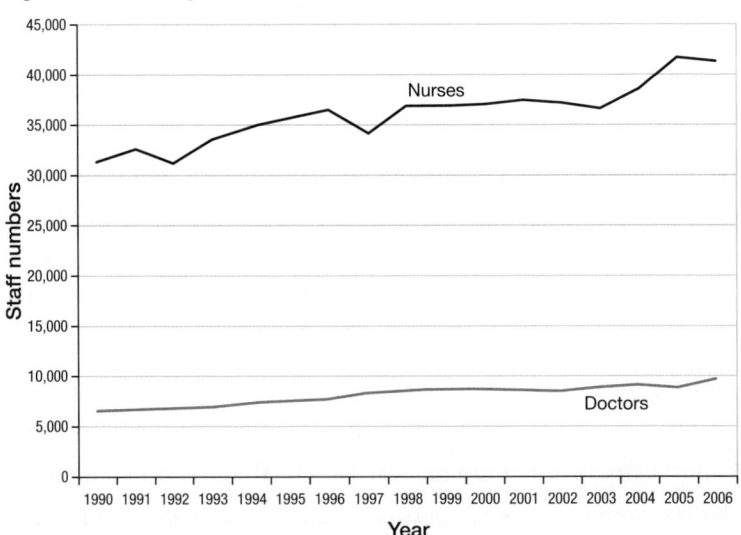

Source   OECD Health Data 2008

The most comprehensive statistics are kept regarding doctors. This is what's been happening to the number of the different kinds of doctor since the year 2000:

Figure 23 **Doctor workforce**

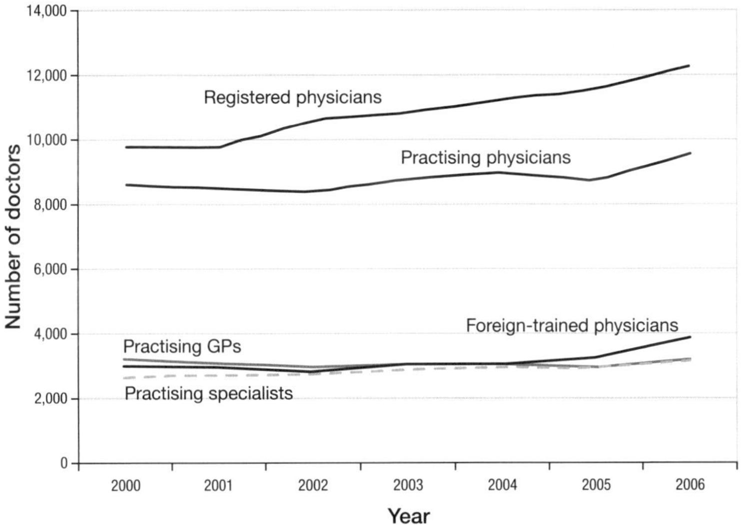

Source   OECD Health Data 2008

The number of registered physicians has been growing steadily. Interestingly, so has the difference between the numbers of those who are registered to practise in New Zealand and those who are actually doing it. Seems there's a whole bunch of doctors out there who have kicked back to feed their chooks or tend the vineyard. GP numbers have been static, while the numbers of other kinds have been growing faster than the general population. Partly, this is because the numbers of foreign-trained doctors have been rising.

So at first glance, the supply of health workers seems generally pretty healthy. But there are concerns about the number of GPs. There were 3,435 practising GPs in 2008, but more than half of these are baby boomers, and will be retiring at precisely the moment the rest of their generation are hobbling toward the surgery door. According to the Health Workforce Advisory Committee,[159] pathology and psychiatry are also facing big issues.

So yes, we appear to have shortages in the system, although in many categories, this is partially offset by the recruitment of foreign-trained doctors. Let's look at the factors that determine the supply of doctors – immigration, training, registration and retention.

Doctors for Africa– or vice versa?

While the media are fond of putting the proportion of foreign doctors working in New Zealand at around 50%, this is actually based on foreign-*born* rather than foreign-trained doctors. The number of foreign-trained doctors has tended to hover around 35% for most of the past twenty years.

Figure 24 **Foreign-trained doctors**

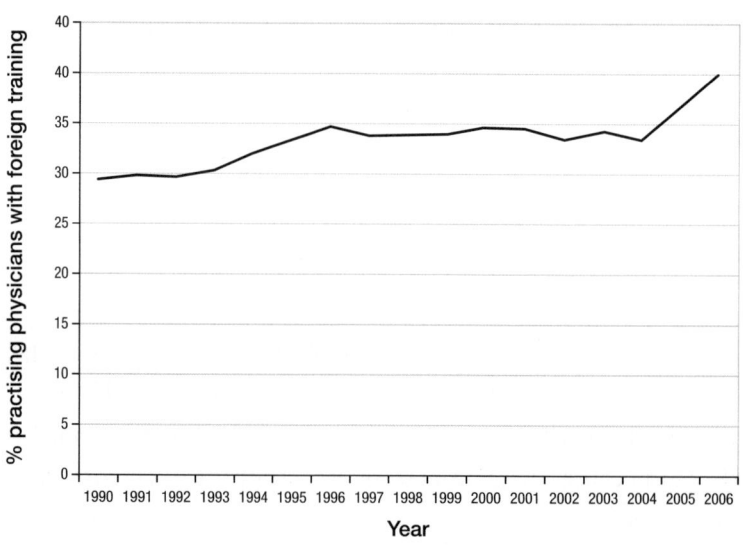

Source   OECD Health Data 2008

The proportion of foreign-trained nurses is lower – at around 24% – but the proportion is growing faster. It doubled between 1994 and 2004.

We've already noted that New Zealand is just another competitor in the global market for healthcare workers, and we're a cash-strapped one at that. Does this mean we're forced to accept second-rate staff from overseas to replace the first-rate staff we train?

In fact, there's no hard evidence to suggest there's anything wrong with our foreign-trained recruits. There's certainly nothing to suggest that foreign-trained doctors are less well trained than the local product, and there's some advantage in the fact that New Zealand didn't have to pay for their education. As we shall see, this training isn't cheap. Anecdotally, however, foreign-trained doctors and nurses may have lower cultural awareness, and can be less effective in the New Zealand context as a result. Foreign-trained doctors also seem to have even itchier feet than their New Zealand-trained counterparts. On average, just over a quarter of foreign-trained doctors are still in the country six years after being hired. Doctors from the United States and the United Kingdom seem most restless, with Asians having the highest rate of retention. But even the rate of retention of Asian-trained doctors – around 50% after six years – lags the 75% of New Zealand-trained doctors retained over the same time period.[160] Many foreign-trained medical staff see New Zealand as a stepping stone toward a career in the United States and Australia, much as locally-trained people do. After all, the United States is the richest system in the world, and the assorted states of Australia have been busily bidding against each other for health workers, pushing salaries up by 50% in the past five years.

Given how expensive it is to recruit foreign-trained health professionals, the low retention rate is a problem, and makes it risky to propose to rely on the overseas supply of trained staff.

You occasionally hear calls for New Zealand to be 'self-sufficient' in its health sector workforce needs. It's unclear what's meant by this. Does it mean replacing locally trained staff with foreigners as quickly as they leave? Does it mean bolting the door from the inside to keep foreigners out, and at the same time, bolting it from the outside to keep our own people from leaving? Either seems impractical at best, impossible at worst and at any rate, undesirable.

In fact, talk of 'self-sufficiency' tends to be xenophobia in disguise. Highly skilled people have always moved around the world, and always will − our own talented doctors and nurses leave; the talented doctors and nurses of other nations arrive. We ought to welcome the latter group, and extend some sort of assistance to help them settle into our sophisticated culture of rugby, racing and beer. But pinching skills from abroad is not a complete answer. We can't neglect training our own.

Training

The other source of new entrants to the workforce is through training our own citizens. New Zealand has tended to train around 285 new doctors per year since 1982. In 2004 this was raised to 325, and in 2007 it was raised again to 365. The Medical Training Board has recommended this number be increased by a further 100. The policy of the National Government is to lift doctor training numbers by 200 to 565.[161] In light of the Medical Training Board recommendations, this seems excessive, given the cost of training doctors, and the very strong likelihood a good proportion of them will take their qualifications and bugger off overseas. Already, about 23% of our nurses and 29% of our doctors are working in other OECD countries.[162] Unless, of course, the National strategy is to train staff faster than they can leave!

It's expensive to train doctors. Back in 2002, the Tertiary Education Commission found that the whole training process cost around $200,000 per doctor, with about 70% ($140,000) being paid by the government and 30% ($60,000) by the student.[163]

Since 2002, the Government has raised its contribution by almost $25,000 per student, although presumably costs have risen, too. And if you're taking a big-picture approach to assessing the cost of medical training, you have to consider that every doctor trained means one more capable person diverted from doing something else. So while we obviously want to meet future demands for medical staff, we could overdo it.

Loan rangers

You don't have to go out of your way to hear medical students – and those concerned at the 'brain drain' – bitching about student loans, which are supposed to contribute to the desire among our best and brightest (doctors and nurses included) taking off for greener pastures. The loans regime has eroded the collegial atmosphere of med schools, we hear, and there's less team spirit. This is said to carry over after graduation: doctors will no longer go the extra mile for their patient if it means staying on beyond their shift. Students no longer feel they owe a debt of obligation to the country for funding their training. They now go for the speciality that will pay off their student loan fastest instead of what the country needs most – hence the shortages in certain areas.

It's frankly hard to see that any of these arguments hold water. The government is still paying the lion's share of the cost – far more toward a doctor's training than towards that of a plumber, for example. Doctors will go on to earn a tidy income, so paying the loans back shouldn't be too much of a problem. And if med students really believe the relationship is one-sided, with the government gone all take, take, take on them by asking them to contribute to the cost of their training, they need only reflect that the nation is getting a pretty poor return on its investment in the third of all doctors who go overseas within 10 years of graduation.

It's difficult to find any means of verifying the anecdotal claims that the contemporary, absolute focus on academic grades means new doctors are less socially conscious, less inquisitive and more risk-averse than in the past. But we can measure the impact of student loans on doctor retention. Student loans were introduced in 1992, so the first year where students graduated bearing the full burden of a student loan was 1998. A slightly higher number of these graduates did head offshore. A year later, however, the effect had vanished without a ripple. Perhaps we alienated the Class of '98 with the introduction of the student loan scheme. Subsequent intakes have proved less emotional about it all.

Nevertheless, the Government has lately seen fit to introduce a voluntary bonding scheme, which will offer generous remuneration subsidies to doctors who commit to staying. It will be interesting to see if it makes any difference in retention, or merely gives more money to doctors who would have stayed anyway. It may help to steer medical graduates into areas where there are shortages – provincial areas, and the problem areas of general practice, psychiatry, pathology, radiology and oncology.

Qualified failure

The other gripe about New Zealand medical training is that it isn't fit for purpose – training hasn't really kept pace with the times, and when it has changed, it has tended to become more academic and less practical. This is particularly alleged of nursing, which used to be learned on the job and supported by a polytechnic course. Now, it's degree-based. Anecdotally, nurses can get a qualification without ever having treated a patient. Naturally, the realities of the hospital experience – the sights, sounds and smells and the raw emotion – are enough to put some of them off their chosen career before they even start.

Some argue that never mind the quality of nurse training: maybe the raw material has deteriorated. Some of our experts observed that twenty years ago, nursing was one of the few career options for talented women. Now there's a lot more choice, and nursing ranks down the list. The standard of nurses is likely to be lower as a result. So what do we do? Restore the community status of the medical professions, such as GPs and nurses, or bring back glass ceilings in other workplaces?

It's harder to argue with the criticism that having 21 DHBs trying to agree on appropriate training standards is near futile. Given this kind of fragmentation, it's little wonder that people fall into the cracks between academic training and on-the-job practical experience. The Medical Training Board has recommended a new body oversee the training interface on behalf of the DHBs, and this seems like an eminently sensible idea.

Closed shops

Health and Community Services staff are the most unionised group of occupations in the country.[164] The Association of Advanced Medical Specialists claim to represent over 90% of senior doctors employed by DHBs.[165] As a result, doctors have considerable clout in their salary demands. This is particularly the case when they are up against the fragmented, disorganised rabble of 21 different DHBs. What's more, only doctors and nurses can really judge whether other doctors and nurses are any good, right? Maybe so, but that gives the medical professions an inordinate amount of power in their workplace, and creates at least the potential that it will be used to anticompetitive ends. After all, one of the easiest ways to keep your salary high would be to restrict the supply of new doctors.

This is precisely what occasionally gets alleged in respect of overseas doctors seeking registration here.[166] The New Zealand Medical Council decides who reaches the necessary standard to be registered to practise in New Zealand. In the past, membership of the NZ Medical Council was restricted to doctors, who were all elected by doctors. The possibility exists that the power to grant or deny registration will be used to regulate the supply of new doctors in a way that favours existing supply and therefore salary levels. Talk about turkeys voting for Christmas!

Does it happen? The Overseas Doctors Association claims that there are 350 foreign-trained doctors in the country at the moment doing low-paid jobs because they can't get registered.[167] Most of us have probably been driven home in a taxi after a night on the town by one of these poor buggers. And certainly successive Labour Health Ministers were concerned enough to attempt to break up the cartel by increasing the number of people appointed rather than elected to the Council. Doctors were, predictably, rather bummed out, but they can't complain too much – the Council still mostly comprises doctors.

Nor, it's been alleged, have the nurses been above such monopolistic behaviour. Overseas nurses are becoming an increasingly important part of the health workforce, yet the Nursing Council recently demanded that foreign-trained nurses undertake an International English language test and achieve a score of 7 or better. That sounds reasonable enough, doesn't it? Until you learn that in order to go to University, the required IELTS score is only 6.[168] The Council declared themselves unhappy with the quality of graduates from the Philippines and ruled that they would only accept four-year qualifications – although many Filipino nurses do a degree before taking up nursing as a second course. So is the Nursing Council merely safeguarding the health of New Zealanders, or does it suit them to starve the system of nurses in order to keep salary levels high?

The rankest example of anticompetitive behaviour in the health sector was revealed in the case of *The Commerce Commission v The Ophthalmological Society of New Zealand & Ors* in 2004. It turned out an Invercargill eye doctor had tried everything in his power to stop Australian doctors coming in and undercutting him, including mounting a concerted effort to block them from being registered to operate in New Zealand. This was an extreme case, but it illustrates what is possible. The use of market power is usually far more subtle. Medical workforce representative groups have a tendency to block proposals for innovation in the roles of health workers. How much of this is because of real safety concerns, and how much is a version of the old 'change of method' walkouts that meatworkers and stevedores staged on a weekly basis in the 1970s?

If doctors are, as they say, solely concerned about safety, why have they resisted all attempts to introduce quality assurance monitoring of doctors, which is an attractive alternative to using the registration process as a barrier to poor practice? Some experts we talked to insisted the registration process should be taken away from the control of doctors altogether.

Hard Docs to keep on the porch

Close to a third of New Zealand-trained doctors are practising overseas or not practising at all 10 years after they graduate. According to the Medical Training Board, if this loss were reduced by as little as 20%, New Zealand *'would gain the equivalent of an extra medical school year intake every 15 years.'*

Terms and conditions are crucial to retention. Pay is a big element, but we've seen that quite apart from the problem of trying to spend it up with the big boys – Australia and the United States – pay increases tend to be absorbed by the existing workforce without necessarily stimulating productivity increases or even more recruitment. One thing we could do with pay scales is to ensure we reward the experience of nurses and doctors. With such a big push on recruitment in recent years, the pay gap between battle-hardened, experienced staff and the fresh-faced recruits has shrunk; some hospitals we visited stopped giving nurses pay increases altogether after five years' experience. And yet the experienced nurse who runs a tight ship, doesn't get flustered and who keeps the doctors' egos in check is the mainstay of the hospital system. So what are we doing to retain them?

When you talk to doctors and nurses, it's pretty clear they derive most of their job satisfaction from the sense they're making a difference, and rather than a handsome pay packet, they're keen to get on with doing the most effective job they can of treating and caring for their patients. So it makes sense to address the circumstances under which they do their job. Our interviews concluded that one of the real ball-breakers for doctors and nurses was the requirement to be 'on call'. The public sector provides a 24-hour emergency service, and this can create all sorts of coverage problems in provincial areas. It also causes problems for staff, particularly as they get older. Being called out at all hours of the night can be a real challenge, particularly when you have family commitments, and when you're expected to show up bright-eyed and bushy-tailed at work the next day. Contracts are improving for doctors, including reductions in on-call hours. Since 2000, average on-call hours for all doctors have fallen by an average of 3.5 hours per week, a reduction of about one third. Specialists used to have almost 17 hours per week on call, but that had dropped to 11 hours by 2008.[169]

Doctors and nurses all complain about increased administration, both the interference in their jobs by management, and the amount of time they are required to push paper instead of pampering or palpating patients. Older doctors will wax lyrical about the old triumvirate of superintendent (doctor), matron (nurse) and bean counter. They argue that this system was simple and kept medical staff engaged in the functioning of hospitals. We'll look at whether we have too many administrators later, but for now let's just focus on the amount of admin that doctors and nurses are asked to do. Staff who operate in both the private and public sectors complain that there is far more paperwork in the latter. A particular area of concern for doctors is safety, which is something of an administrative Kinleith. It seems there are many different and overlapping procedures for dealing with breaches in patient safety: there are forms to be filled in for ACC, the Health and Disability Commissioner, internal hospital and DHB processes, the Medical Council, select committees, sentinel reporting and, on occasion, intense interest from the media. In theory, Kiwi doctors should be better off than overseas – they can't be sued for treatment injuries in New Zealand thanks to the existence of ACC. In theory (again), this should create an environment in which people can freely admit mistakes and work together to eliminate them in the future. But doctors we talked to felt the sheer number of safety audits conducted after the most trifling mistake still creates a risk-averse attitude. This probably also inflates costs and leads to the provision of unnecessary treatment. Some doctors we met even said they'd rather be sued, because at least under that system you can insure yourself against the cost and rely on the legal process to run interference with the media.

Plenty of medical staff we talked to enjoy the work they do and prefer to get on with it without distractions. One surgeon we talked to, who has both public and private practices, contrasted the efficiency of the private sector – where support staff organised his entire day and made sure his patients were ready so he could spend the maximum amount of time operating – with the public sector. Here, he had little administrative support and, worse, a considerable administrative workload. He had to attend meetings and read and comment on documents. Even when he was supposed to be performing operations, he would often be kept waiting while the next patient was organised, or he'd be stood down because the operating theatre had been commandeered for an emergency. He found the private sector far more satisfying because he spent much more of his time doing what he wanted to do – using his training to help people. This is what the latest report on senior doctors in New Zealand means when it recommends that the public system work to ensure doctors have access to the 'space, tools and support...' they need.[170]

A plague of locums – the demand for medical staff

We've got more doctors and nurses than ever before, even when adjusting for population. But other countries we like to compare ourselves to have more than us, and even they aren't satisfied with their staffing levels. Meanwhile, newspaper headlines scream about dangerous staffing shortages in our local DHB. How can this be?

That there are genuine shortages in the system at large is evident in the emergence of a lucrative market for locums – the health sector version of a temp. Some hospitals lack full-time junior doctors or other staff to cover all their shifts, let alone holidays, sickness or maternity leave. According to the New Zealand Herald, some provincial hospitals have up to 50% of their positions vacant.[171] Locums cover these shortfalls – we heard of some units with locums comprising up to 75% of their staff. Between 2002 and 2008, spending on locum staff grew by 115%.[172] This rise has been even bigger (180%) in the five smallest provincial DHBs, which employ disproportionate numbers of locums. Like any temp, you pay a bit more for a flexible worker, sometimes up to double the usual rate. Trouble is, locums now find it so easy to get work whenever they want it that it has become a viable and lucrative career choice. Why bother going to the effort and expense of specialising when you can earn the same amount plying your trade as a locum junior doctor?

Since workforce numbers haven't fallen, clearly workforce 'shortages' arise from increased demand for staff. As you'll recall, this is because we demand far more treatment than our forbears for the same conditions. This trend is likely to continue in the future. There are also the problems of supplier-induced demand

and overtreatment.

There are other factors at work, too. These include moonlighting in the private sector, health workforce bargaining and workforce responsibilities.

A bit on the side

If you spend enough time in New Zealand's public and private hospitals, a lot of the faces start looking pretty familiar. It is fairly common for doctors, particularly surgeons, to work in both. For those of us accustomed to having one full-time job, this may seem a little weird, but it's pretty common in the medical profession.

Doctors' contracts have become more generous in recent years as we struggle to compete with burgeoning offshore pay packets. We pay more and we offer more time off for study and training. Many doctors opt to keep their eye in by working for private clinics. The pocket money isn't bad, either.

There's a potential conflict of interest here. If your patient in the public sector lets slip that they're capable of paying for the procedure, why not steer them in the direction of your private practice? And once you've got the taste, why bother trying to be effective and efficient in the public sector at all? Better, surely, to keep your public list waiting long enough to spook the cashed-up over to the private sector.

We understand from our conversations that this happens – particularly in highly specialised areas where doctors have more control over the market – but does it happen enough to cause the system problems? Most of our respondents pointed out that the behaviour of doctors is governed by fairly stringent moral codes, which stop this sort of abuse. Doctors are supposed to declare any interest when referring a patient, and to offer a choice. Yeah, well, real estate agents are supposed to act only in the vendor's best interests, too. There are no studies comparing the productivity of doctors in the public and private sectors; even if it could be shown that there was a difference, could anyone say for sure it's the fault of the doctor rather than the system around them?

In the private sector, for example, doctors are rewarded for performing procedures. In the public sector, most are on a salary and there's generally no incentive to be as productive as possible. This and the added bureaucracy doctors must wrestle in the public sector meant that they generally get far more done in their private practice. Most surgeons we talked to were frustrated by this: they enjoy operating and want to do it as much as possible.

There may well be benefits to the public sector hospitals from the practice of moonlighting. It allows doctors to supplement their public sector income, and thus may prevent their skills being lost to the public sector – or even to the country – altogether. In sparsely populated areas, working in both the public and private sectors can increase the amount of available work for specialists, making it viable for them to locate in provincial areas. Not that you'll see ophthalmologists flocking to Opotiki: poor rural areas won't support the private practice opportunities that affluent rural areas will.

In summary, then, most of the experts we talked to felt that the practice of doctors moonlighting in the private sector is an evil, but probably a necessary one. And perhaps the answer to whatever problems might arise from it is to emulate the best practices from the private sector in the public, so that highly trained medical staff get to spend the maximum amount of time doing what they love to do in the public system, too. The moves that some DHBs have recently made toward establishing units dedicated to elective surgery – so that there's no more 'gazumping' of elective surgery by emergency ops – is a step in the right direction.

DHBs – where everyone gets a bargain

Curiously, in light of what we've been discussing, improving the pay and conditions of medical staff has actually *contributed* to staffing shortages. Contracts have become a lot more focused on work-life balance, with improved pay, reduced hours on call, the aforementioned 'training leave' and reduced hours overall. So we're paying doctors more, and they're working less! Economists are familiar with this phenomenon, and call it 'a backward bending labour supply curve'. You'd probably call it chilling out once you feel you've earned enough.

Historically, junior doctors put in big hours to provide a basic level of medical cover. Junior doctors these days work just over 50 hours per week on average.[173] Luxury! Older doctors talk about doing 80-hour weeks with more than a hint of grim nostalgia, as though it were some form of initiation rite their modern counterparts are too soft to endure. 80 hours! Aye, tell that t'young folk these days, they'll never believe ya.

Of course, softer junior doctors means you need more of them simply to provide a basic level of medical cover, particularly in small provincial hospitals. And not only is the present-day crop soft, they're stroppy, too: older doctors lament that there's no willingness among junior doctors to help out when there are staff shortages, unless they're paid at the locum rate. This can have a catastrophic effect on a small provincial hospital. To provide a service, it needs to have a doctor available 24 hours a day, 7 days a week. The key constraint is after-hours cover. In the past, when men were real men and women were mostly nurses, junior doctors worked 80 hours a week and napped in hospital beds; the unit may have needed three junior doctors to cover a service over the whole week. Now working hours are less and on-call availability is limited. You may now need at least five doctors working full-time in order to cover the night shifts. Across a whole hospital, that's a lot more staff. During the day, some teams are now tripping over each other without enough work to do, while at night they are stretched to the limit. Conditions were probably excessively harsh in the past, and who knows how many mistakes were made by junior doctors in the 80th hour of that particular working week. But to a large extent, the entire system was built around the exploitation of trainee doctors.

Diminished workforce responsibilities

The health sector of the future will demand a very different type of health worker. They will need to be more generalist and holistic, able to work as part of a team dealing with the burgeoning numbers of patients with chronic diseases. They will need to be able to work in partnership with the patients themselves, empowering them to treat themselves and manage their own illnesses...

This touchy-feely vision of the future is a long way from the current reality. If anything, we seem to be heading in the other direction. Many current health workers are protective of their roles and resistant to potential change, and if anything, doctors are becoming increasingly specialised. 'General surgery' for example, has become increasingly broken down into sub-specialities. Some nurses complain that doctors still stand on the old hierarchical ceremonies, rather than pitching in as team players. Patients are not always empowered – on the contrary, many are so unengaged as to refuse to take the treatment that they are prescribed.

Hutt Valley DHB summer student programme

For four weeks in January 2009, six 2nd and 3rd year students from Otago Medical School spent time in the Hutt Valley DHB seeing how different parts of the health system worked. Their visits were carefully chosen to demonstrate how modern healthcare should ideally be delivered – in multidisciplinary teams with a focus on prevention. The students spent time with GPs, nurses, physiotherapists and occupational therapists and got firsthand experience of a hospital operating theatre and a Maori community provider as well as doing time on the ambulances.

The purpose of the programme was to give future doctors a broader perspective on healthcare before they became focused on their area of speciality. In particular, the future doctors saw how primary care integrates with the hospital: they got to see the medical journey for the patient right through the health system. This seems to have worked, judging by some of the participant feedback: *'statistics on a page do not hit home until you are sitting in someone's decrepit house and hearing their story and you understand so many people have no one or nothing...'* and *'Being a doctor includes more than interaction between doctor and patient – [it] includes nurses, physios, primary and secondary, PHOs...'.*

This increasing sub-specialisation is exacerbating the demand for doctors, and in provincial areas, a whole new team of staff may be needed to deliver a service where none was needed before.

Partly, the problem is due to medical culture. Kudos in the doctor world consists very much of your degree of 'specialisation'. Bugger being an all-rounder: doctors prefer to be the cutting-edge scientist who delves deeply into a new area. Our best and brightest are encouraged to specialise; show them a spleen, say, and they'll feel right at home. Ask them to take a patient's medical history and they'll run for the hills. This has been an increasing trend throughout the rise of modern medicine. In 1961, over 50% of practising doctors were GPs, but by 2006 this had fallen to 33%.[174]

Partly, this is driven in its turn by the way in which remuneration happens in the private sector, where the bias is towards procedures. Never mind that just as much skill (if not more) is needed to get a good diagnosis of your problem, and to give you a comprehensive understanding of treatment options: the surgeon who offers you an operation is offering you something concrete and for a settled price. You're consequently far more likely to shell out to have a fibre-optic cable stuck down your throat so you can see your ulcers being treated on the big screen (with the optional DVD available for just $50 more) rather than have a pleasant chat about how to cope with your complex, rare but ultimately untreatable condition. And because you won't shell out just for a chat, a doctor without a procedure is doomed to eking out a six-figure salary, rather than coining the seven digits their mates in ophthalmology can command.

Doctors spend a long time learning how to do what they do, and along the way, they make a large investment in their own self-belief. It's galling for most of us to be told that someone with far less training than us could do just as good a job (although it's so often true). But occasionally, doctors need to take care to ensure their resistance to innovations in their field has to do with patient safety rather than mere professional pique or the territorial instinct that marks out restrictive trade practices.

It's been proposed, for example, that nurses or even trained technicians could perform some routine procedures that currently require (at their insistence) fully qualified doctors at the wheel. New Zealand has one of the highest rates of colon cancer in the world, and recently proposed universal screening for colon cancer. Trouble is, there aren't enough gastroenterologists in the country to carry out the number of colonoscopies required to make it work. Indeed, there weren't enough to cover demand *before* the screening programme was announced.[175] The solution? Train more gastroenterologists, say the gastroenterologists. But is that the only way? In Canada and the US, colonoscopies have been undertaken by nurses for many years, and in fact, there's reason to believe they're done better because the personnel involved specialise in the procedure.

Many modern procedures, like colonoscopies, are so technologically assisted that they could be performed by anyone with a moderate aptitude on the X-Box. What need, then, for the six years' worth of training in the details of how the whole human body works? Doctors would still be needed to make the diagnosis – which is where their skills are really applied – and to oversee operations in case things went wrong. But in this model, they would become far more like the builder who paces about the site overseeing his army of apprentices and subbies who are doing all the actual measuring, hammering and sawing.

There's little chance of this kind of lateral thinking being applied to the problem of staff shortages while the doctors have a say in it – unless, of course, sheer necessity compels it. General Practitioners in some areas are entitled to undertake minor surgery, usually trained and overseen by specialists through 'clinical networks'. This has the added benefit of inducing doctors in an area to interact, lowering the barriers between primary and hospital care, and it also creates the opportunity to intervene at the earliest possible stage of an illness (as where a GP can not only detect, but also remove a skin cancer). A good example of this approach is the ACC scheme of GPs with 'a Special Interest'. Due to a lack of orthopaedic surgeons in certain areas, ACC employs GPs with advanced skills and training in this area. The GPs assist with the diagnosis of disorders and the creation of treatment plans for non-urgent patients, and are given access to diagnostic services to help them. Normally, GPs must refer patients to a specialist for some diagnostic services. This approach has been trialled in three regions – Hawkes Bay, Dunedin and Invercargill – with promising results. It's surely worth rolling out on the national scale.

Heal thyself

Devolving some of the responsibilities incumbent on – or jealously reserved by – doctors onto nurses or technicians is one area of innovation that will doubtless need to be explored as personnel shortages become more acute. Nurses may well become key carers in cases of chronic illness, where there is a need to coordinate different treatments. And we may have to go further still, with much of the responsibility for managing treatments assumed by patients themselves. This approach aims to create 'expert' patients – after all, patients are the expert in their own lives, and will know what works best for them. Naturally, patients need to be informed about the condition to make this work. But more than this, they need to be given the skills to manage their behaviour consistent with their goal (for example, to take the drugs or stick to the diet). Teaching these skills takes additional time and effort, but can save money and improve outcomes over the long term.[176] It may even help address the growing hunger out there for more and more treatment.

Evidence suggests that 'expert' patients don't necessarily need to be trained about their condition by health professionals.[177] Similarly, case managers for chronic patients don't always need to be health sector workers – part of their role could be picked up by other specialities (such as dietitians or personal trainers) or even 'peer mentors'. Peer mentoring links a patient with someone who suffers from or who has suffered from the same condition and has learned to manage it. Peer mentors can empathise with the patient, do some of the hand-holding that some people expect from doctors and nurses, and can make sure communication is effective both ways between doctor and patient.

Summary

In summary, then, there are escalating demands on our health system. While supply can and will be increased over time, it is never likely to fully satiate this demand. This continued pressure will hopefully spur innovation in the way healthcare is delivered, but don't count on it, when there is so much vested interest in the way.

Chapter 8

+OO MANY CHIEFS, NOT ENOUGH INDIANS?

'Bureaucracy is the art of making the possible impossible'
Javier Pascual Salcedo.

Healthcare can be a lot tougher to run than many other industries. After all, it's the medical team (in consultation with the patient) who make decisions about what the appropriate treatment is, and this determines what costs are being incurred. Consequently, medical teams wield considerable power and responsibility – not only over our health and well-being, but over how they spend our tax dollars, too.

For this reason, the effective functioning of the health system is almost entirely dependent upon a good relationship between administrators and staff. Too much power on one side often leads to problems. The National government, bless them, notoriously tried giving all the power to professional administrators in the 1990s. And recently, the New South Wales Government experimented with handing over full control of their hospitals to the doctors. Those hospitals have since run out of money, and couldn't afford to make salary payments or purchase basic antibiotics.

While further change to our health system seems inevitable if it is to meet the demands of the future, it was clear from our interviews that staff are understandably fatigued from two decades of change already. Time is needed to build up a relationship of trust between administrators and medical staff, and perhaps that time is best used to map out a future course of action that everyone can buy into.

To listen to workers in the public health system, you'd think administrators were a kind of infestation. Their numbers have got way out of hand, it's argued, and they're a waste of precious resources, anyway. But as evil as you may regard administration to be, it's a necessary one. You don't want doctors and nurses charged with booking appointments, chasing up patients, ensuring the health system runs to a budget and doing the reporting upon which we decide whether we're getting value for our money. These are nonetheless vital tasks, and they do require some specialised skills of their own. That's why we have administrators.

Have we gone overboard with professional management? Perhaps we did in the 1990s, but then again, such coarse indicators as we have of efficiency – patient Average Length of Stay is one – suggest that things weren't run particularly efficiently under the old unholy trinity of Medical Super, Matron and Accountant, either. That system was as prone to dysfunction as anything we've devised since.

So it seems that like so much else in life, a fine balance must be struck. We don't want doctors and nurses spending all their time running the show, but we need their input to decision-making.

As for the proposition that administration is absorbing more of our health dollars than it used to, it's hard to test. Prior to 1980, few if any records were kept to show how money was spent and what outcomes were secured as a result. But the patchy data that we do have suggests that spending on administration actually *fell* following Labour's 1988 reforms of the public health service. It's difficult to tell what happened after the National reforms of the 1990s, as health administration data disappears again. However, over the period 1992 to 2006, health administrative spending grew and by 2006 was back above the 1987 levels in real terms.

Given quite a lot of admin funding went into implementing reforms, the rate of growth seems quite mild. From 1987 to 2006, health administration spending more or less matched GDP growth, and as health spending more generally has grown far faster than GDP, administration has actually *fallen* as a proportion of total health spending, with most of the decrease likely to be attributable to the earliest reforms in 1988. Since 1992, administration has been steady at around 4% of the total health budget. This is about average for the OECD, given the size of our economy. About one dollar in every 300 we earn as a country goes into healthcare administration. This is a long way from the US, where the figure is one in 90. It's only when you compare our administrative spend with other countries with a comparable reliance on their public health system that we look expensive. Even so, administration hardly looks like the wealth-destruction machine that embittered medical staff would have us believe it is. Bureaucrats in Wellington are certainly not the real cost driver, as a recent report pointed out: *'if the Ministry of Health were removed [in September], its equivalent cost would be back in time for Christmas dinner'.*[178]

This doesn't mean that there is no waste in the health system, and certainly doesn't absolve administrators, either. Time and motion studies conducted by Counties Manukau DHB indicate 15-20% of staff time is wasted, and this can be reduced to about 5%. This means each nurse could potentially spend another hour with patients per shift – a bit like the country having another 4,000 nurses! This is possible if administrators work with hospital staff to ensure that systems are set up to help doctors and nurses do a quality job.

Let's start by assuming administration costs are a little high and looking at why this might be. Then we'll look at quality and efficiency more broadly.

Think local, act parochial – the DHB/PHO madness

The prime candidate for the title of most wasteful deployment of administrative resources is the health system's expression of parochialism, namely the District Health Board/Primary Health Organisation system. We've already seen how our individual sense of entitlement places undue pressure on the health system. It turns out that its equivalent at the community level does just about does the same amount of damage.

Let's take a sentimental journey through the history of the New Zealand health administration numbers:

- Pre 1988 – 30 Health Boards
- 1988-1992 – 14 Area Health Boards
- 1993-1998 – 23 Crown Health Enterprises (that deliver healthcare) and 4 Regional Health Authorities (which did the purchasing on behalf of the government)
- 1998-2000 – 23 Hospital and Health Services and 1 Health Funding Authority
- 2000-present – 21 District Health Boards (DHBs)
- 2002-present – 80+ Primary Health Organisations.

We've previously alleged in this book that the prime motivation for the reorganisation of health decision-making since 2000 was political. The National government's failed health reforms had been desperately unpopular, so the Clark-led Labour Government that followed saw a golden opportunity to win brownie points with the electorate. The easiest way to reverse the funder/provider split that was at the heart of National's programme was to do the bare minimum – change the 23 HHSs already in existence into funders as well as providers. This had the attractive spin-off of palming off the unpopularity that comes with making difficult funding decisions in the health area onto the new District Health Boards.

It's pretty hard to find any other justification, or any evidence of benefits arising from Labour's actions. There are now 21 District Health Boards – still way too many organisations for a country of four million people – which vary in size from the West Coast (with a population of 31,000) to Waitemata (482,000). Their existence clearly has nothing to do with service quality or economies of scale. And it's pretty hard to be convinced by the rhetoric that the DHB structure makes decision-makers more 'locally accountable'. When communities first acquired the right to vote for the membership of their DHBs in 2001, only half of us bothered to fill in the postal vote. This has since fallen to 43% in 2007 – about the same as most other local elections. Once the Board is elected, what local accountability is there? Their real accountability, as stated in legislation, is to the Minister of Health, not voters or the community. Besides, some of these so-called democratic decisions are made behind closed doors.

And anyway, is putting decision-making within reach of interest groups really such a good idea for our healthcare funding? Because of all the blue rinses in the waiting rooms, Grey Power has got all the DHB boards by the short and curlies, and they use this power to squeeze DHBs whenever they don't churn out enough new hips and knees for the fading.

So what value do District Health Boards add? Doctors decide who gets treated, although pressure groups can bring down politically motivated decrees as well. The Boards can hardly be regarded as fiercely independent champions of local need against the meddling of central government. Historical spending patterns, dictates from the Ministry of Health and political pressure to keep certain hospitals or units running largely determine where DHB money goes. Some former Board members we talked to complain that these pressures leave very little room for local flexibility. DHBs are obliged to produce a local 'Health Needs Assessment' that's supposed to identify local needs and guide investment decisions. These reports generally become expensive doorstops, and have little impact on decisions.[179] Even where they do have the elbow room to make a difference, some experts we talked to were of the opinion that DHB Board members often had conflicts of interest.

So what value can be placed on 'local accountability'? If we're being honest, doesn't it all just boil down to 'our DHB Board bloody well better keep our local hospital open'? For while they're charged with addressing the local health needs – broadly considered – of their catchment, a concern about local hospital services underlies practically all the thinking and decision-making of the DHBs, just as a wilful blindness, born of political expediency, to the obvious need for rationalisation of the national hospital system prompted Labour to saddle us with the DHB system in the first place.

In fact, far from being merely valueless, the DHB model actually leads to huge inequities in the volume and quality of care around the country. Many DHBs simply lack the scale to be viable, to maintain the range of services that their population would expect to have access to. But just try suggesting that the money spent keeping a third-rate hospital open would be better spent on initiatives designed to improve overall community health! It's surprising how quickly small-town New Zealanders can lay their hands on pitchforks when they need to form an angry mob. It's all part of a narrow mindset that is intent on the urgent at the expense of the important – we feel something is being done when bodies are being scraped up from the bottom of the cliff, but we're anxious if it's decided to hire fewer ambulance crews but more fencers to erect the safety barrier at the top. But cheer up, it's not just us: the preoccupation with providing for emergency treatment over and above more effective preventive measures is a world-wide phenomenon that has been labelled the 'rule of rescue'.[180] It causes headaches for healthcare decision-makers around the world, because it is a major obstacle to rational prioritisation.

In order to provide 24/7 service, a DHB requires its hospital to have a minimum number of staff. This usually means that a small traditional hospital has more staff than are needed in a normal day, in order to provide a skeleton staff overnight. So we'd expect their costs to go up, and if that's not matched by a larger budget, we'd expect a reduction in the DHB's ability to provide other services. With all those people you have on to meet emergency demand, you'd find yourself with a whole bunch of people who were surplus to your normal day operations, so you'd constantly be on the hunt to find them stuff to do. How about minor, routine, elective procedures? So we'll need to make sure we employ general surgeons who can cope with a range of mundane stuff.

Overall, then, you'd expect provincial DHBs to have higher costs, fewer services and a high throughput in the range of routine treatments they can offer. They are typically staffed by surgeons with more general skills, so to keep themselves busy, they'll offer more run-of-the-mill elective procedures.

And what do you know? That's exactly what's happening. Let's have a look at DHB resources, service range and treatment levels in turn.

DHB resources

The Ministry of Health divvies up our health budget and gives most of it to DHBs on the basis of their population. They then make a bunch of adjustments for various factors including rurality, tourist volumes and population make-up (in terms of age and ethnicity). The effect of these adjustments is shown in the graph below, which depicts which DHBs get a lower or higher allocation of the total funding pot than you would expect if funding were allocated purely on the basis of their population. If you are above the line, you get more; if you're below, you get less:

Figure 25 **Postcode lottery: health funding winners and losers**

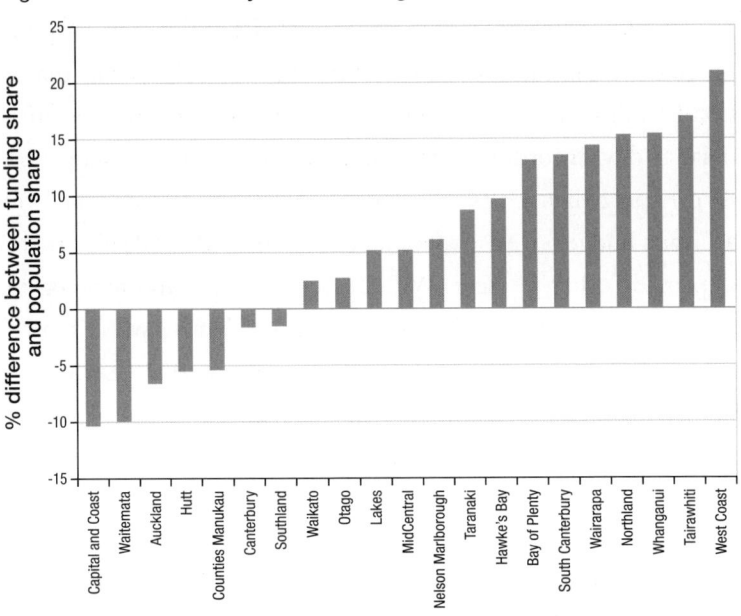

Source   MOH population based funding formula

Spot the cross-subsidisation! Sure, it costs more to offer comprehensive health services in provincial areas, but how much more? How much should the citizens of Waitemata and Wellington dole out so that Greymouth can keep its local hospital running?

And here we arrive at the critical issue. On what basis is it decided to keep a small hospital running? Is it merely the threat of political unpopularity, or is there a rational basis? How much must a hospital cost in terms of QALYs (quality adjusted life years) sacrificed elsewhere before it makes no sense to keep it open?

The simple fact is that a number of these small provincial hospitals are too small to be viable, and staff don't want to work there. The two areas with the lowest numbers of doctors per head of population are Wairarapa and West Coast,[181] despite having two of the highest per capita funding levels. The experts we interviewed commented that hospitals in these areas don't have enough work to attract quality senior doctors, or to justify providing the latest facilities. So why would junior doctors want to work there? Consequently, these areas are increasingly at the mercy of expensive locums and overseas doctors – over half of the doctors at West Coast DHB are foreign-trained and their spending on locums is eight times the national average.[182]

Nor does chucking extra cash at provincial hospitals improve their situation. It turns out that the biggest deficits run by New Zealand DHBs are by those who have money taken off them to fund the provincial hospital subsidies (as you'd expect), *and* by those that receive them – i.e. provincial hospitals themselves. The only areas that don't have significant deficits are the ones in the middle – average-sized DHBs with budgets that match their population. There's a message here somewhere.

Range of services – breathe easy(?) the DHBs are in charge!
Provincial DHBs struggle to provide a full range of services. Let's look at one of New Zealand's big health problems, respiratory diseases, as an example. According to the Asthma and Respiratory Foundation, New Zealand *'has one of the highest prevalence rates of asthma in the world, with asthma occurring in about 15% to 20% of children and adults and affecting at least 600,000 people.'*[183] The economic cost of this disease is over $800 million per year. Similarly COPD (chronic obstructive pulmonary disease – an umbrella term for lung problems developed as a result of tobacco smoking) is *'ranked 2nd in men and 5th in women with regards to its health impact, is the 4th leading cause of death after cancer, heart disease and stroke and is estimated to cost up to $192m in direct healthcare costs each year.'*[184]

If you bundle all respiratory diseases together, they're a bigger cause of mortality than heart disease and cancer.[185] Overseas evidence suggests this group of diseases is also one area where healthcare can have the biggest bang-for-buck impact, with a cost of around $10-15,000 per quality adjusted life year saved.[186] Diabetes, by contrast, is considerably more expensive.

So respiratory problems are a big problem here, and it's relatively cost-effective to do something about it. New Zealand should have a world-class approach to respiratory diseases, right?

Turns out respiratory care in some DHBs needs to be put on an iron lung. According to a recent report in the New Zealand Medical Journal, fewer than half of them comply with the minimum standards of care for these conditions. Staff numbers are inadequate, people are not getting the tests they need, and there's huge geographic variability in quality of care – in some areas we prescribe *seven times* the amount of ventilation equipment for respiratory disorders than in others. Most of those falling short of the minimum standard are in the smaller, provincial DHBs. For patients living in underperforming DHB areas, the effects of postcode lottery can be quite literally breathtaking.

Supplier-induced demand, aka bored provincial doctor syndrome
Doctors are intelligent, motivated people. They are highly trained, and enjoy doing what they're trained to do. But when doctors don't have enough to do, they tend to find problems where there are none. Oh-oh! Supplier-induced demand, again.

Small provincial hospitals need to hire more doctors than they really require during the 9-5 week in order to provide a minimum level of service out-of-hours. These poor doctors get itchy scalpel fingers. And the DHB, bless its cotton socks, needs to have something to show for its money, so Dr Finlay's hard case book really gets let loose here. So we should expect to see more treatments in the range of services that are offered in small provincial areas. And *voilà!* Three of the four DHBs with the highest surgical intervention rates (in other words the percentage of their population they slice and dice) were West Coast, Whanganui and South Canterbury.[187] But rather than deliver according to patient need, provincial hospitals seem to over-treat people for the conditions where they have the capacity, and under-treat for everything else. It's a source of inefficiency, and hard to justify if you're applying rational principles of prioritisation.

In short, then, **DHB** parochialism is keeping uneconomic hospitals open in remote provincial areas. This is costing urban areas, as they're cross-subsidising their country cousins. Meanwhile, it's those very urban areas that most need to invest in order to prepare for the future strains of population growth and the ageing population bulge. This tension renders small provincial areas losers too – their level of treatment across the board leaves much to be desired, because the DHB is frantically trying to keep the hospital open. When you ask people if they'd like their local hospital (or a unit therein) closed, most people predictably say 'no'. But this is an incomplete question. The honest question would be: do you want substandard services at your local hospital (butcher), or would you prefer to travel a bit and have the best? Or even better, how about never needing a hospital at all? A healthcare provider in rural US, Geisinger, spends less on hospitals and more on technology that monitors people's health within their own homes, which picks up problems before they happen. This initiative has reduced hospital admissions by 20%.[188]

Primary health organisations
The duplications and solecisms in the DHB model are one thing. Another present from the Labour-led government was the plethora of Primary Health Organisations that form yet another layer of bureaucracy in the system. We've formerly praised Helen Clark's government for the sensible decision to prioritise primary healthcare. But we find we have to draw a line here – not to pooh-pooh the PHOs totally but just to point out that again, there's too many of them.

Primary Health Organisations are groups of GPs, nurses and other health professionals (such as pharmacists, physios and midwives) who purchase or deliver healthcare services in the community to their enrolled populations. PHOs are paid on the basis of the number of people enrolled, rather than per visit to a GP (as was historically the case). This was intended to encourage them to prevent problems amongst their patients rather than merely wait till they presented and treat them.

Why do we need PHOs as well as DHBs? Because DHBs are hospital-centric, and GPs are stubborn buggers who are fiercely protective of their right to self-determination. PHOs were seen as the best way of getting GPs together. To create them, the Government allowed existing organisations or groups of GPs to bid for the right to deliver primary care to their enrolled population – and the more people they enrolled on their books, the more money they got.

Labour set up an open application process, and initially PHOs got more money if they had a high proportion of Maori and Pacific people or if they operated in poorer communities. This proved to be an incentive for clinics operating in poor areas to set up on their own as PHOs. Everywhere else, GPs got together in fairly large PHOs so they could capture economies of scale in administration. It would, with the benefit of hindsight, have been a better idea to get DHBs to work with the GP groups that were already in existence (Independent Practitioner Associations). How simple would that have been! That would have avoided creating over 80 PHOs with huge variations in size (the biggest four cover 30% of our population, while the smallest 44 average less than 13,000 people each) and corresponding variations in approach. Evaluations show the big PHOs are great at organisation and strategy while the small ones are great at community-oriented delivery.[189] While some of the innovation is great, the sheer number of PHOs makes getting things done in primary care really tough.

Quality, safety & efficiency

Another big complaint about administration we heard through our interviews with doctors was that quality and safety concerns are suffocating public sector treatment. Presumably these processes exist for a reason: so how big an issue is safety? If there *are* safety problems, what are the causes and what's the best way of dealing with them?

Some people have a fear of flying, although the risk of dying in an air accident is one in 8.5 million.[190] That's pretty low, but boy, do you hear about it when a plane goes down.

Comparatively few people, by contrast, have a fear of submitting to an operation, which is surprising when you consider the risk. In 2007/08, DHBs reported 258 people were involved in an *'adverse clinical event that was actually or potentially preventable'*, (a nice way to say, 'butchered') with 76 dying during or shortly afterwards.[191] Before you get too stressed, this is out of 900,000 hospital discharges – a risk of about one in 3,500, the same as in planes that cross Iran. But this is just the *reported* figures. As we saw in Chapter Two, work by academic Peter Davis suggests that up to one in every eight hospital patients are affected by adverse events, with up to two in 100 serious events where the person is killed or disabled by unintended treatment injuries.[192] That would mean there are over 100,000 adverse events in hospitals every year, 9,000 of them serious. Compared to this level of problems, the 1,295 complaints to the Health and Disability Commissioner in 2007/08 is relatively low and the 258 incidents reported by DHBs is even lower. There's evidence that medical staff don't report minor mistakes that might otherwise go unnoticed.[193] Thus, the majority of problems go unnoticed, or are simply accepted by the public as part of the natural order of things. This is pretty common – in the US, people are more likely to sue their doctor for being rude than incompetent.[194]

After reading these figures, you may be wondering if you'd be better off heading to Oz next time you get need an operation. Before you go, you need to know that our rate of 'adverse events' is about the international average, and of course, if you're heading to Oz, you're assuming the additional risk of an 'adverse aviation event'.

Some of the risk that we submit to every time we go under the knife (or drugs, or radiation therapy) arises from the fact that trainee doctors must learn on the job. It's all very well to console ourselves that we learn by our mistakes: that's cold comfort if your trainee pilot makes a mistake when he's putting the airliner down, or your trainee surgeon cuts off the wrong thing. Indeed, this cold comfort is all that's available to the countless deceased patients to whom we owe so much of the state of modern medicine, as the delightful vignette below shows.

The aviation industry confronts the fact that mistakes by learner-drivers kill passengers: it trains pilots for adverse events on a simulator and checks them out on simulators from time to time even once they've graduated. Simulators exist in medicine also, but not for every known procedure. Even where they are available, they're seldom used, and there's presently no system for monitoring a surgeon or doctor's quality. In fact, the rather draconian safety reviews that kick in when a mistake is made is the only check on our doctors' performance that the system has.

Heart failure

For a long time heart surgery was considered the final frontier of medicine – some doctors thought attempting it was madness. Their standpoint was vindicated by the initial forays into experimental heart surgery, which was littered with gore and corpses. Without brave and desperate volunteers to operate on (most of whom would have died soon anyway), heart surgery would never have developed. Initially, heart surgery was little more than doctors groping around blind inside a still beating heart, trying to find and clear blockages with a finger, or quickly sew up holes in the heart. Many of the pioneers of heart surgery gave up when the body count simply got too high.

The American Dwight Harken was one of these pioneers and he nearly quit after six of his first ten patients died. After the last failure he went home and literally hid in his bed. The President of the Heart Foundation pestered him day after day to return to work but he refused to, as he put it 'kill any more people'. The President finally motivated him with the line 'you must have learnt something from those six disasters'. What an encouraging fellow – anyway it must have worked because he coaxed him back to work. Only one of his next 15 patients died. Over time, Dwight and the other surgeons improved with practice, and so did the techniques and survival rates. Nowadays heart surgery, while still a major procedure, is a fairly standard part of the health system. None of us would wish Dwight had stayed in his bed and given up, but none of us would have wanted to be one of his early guinea pigs either.[195]

Doctors generally resist guidelines or formal quality monitoring, and medical commentator James Le Fanu believes there are cultural reasons for this. Again, there's an analogy with the aviation industry. Early surgeons and doctors, like aviators in the early days of flight, tended to be the gung-ho alpha males, flying by the seat of their pants, resourceful enough to improvise when things started going haywire. Doctors also argue that any attempt to implement procedures and guidelines inevitably leads to overtreatment, as doctors hide behind guidelines to reduce the risk of a damaging external review. However, no doctor can be expected to keep up with international best practice for every treatment – a GP would need to read for 27 hours each day just to keep up with the latest health research and development. The real issue is getting the guidelines right – they need to stick to evidenced, cost-effective treatment and leave room for customisation where applicable.

Doctors prefer to self-regulate performance through peer review. This is fine, but only if there's a system of monitoring and quality control. Above all, those who make mistakes must be prepared to report them, be accountable for their outcomes and work to improve their performance. After all, a conscientious willingness to address mistakes has often led to the development of new procedures. So both sides are a little bit right – on the one hand, we need more streamlined safety procedures, but doctors can't keep our confidence just by brushing off safety concerns with 'Trust me, I know what I'm doing', either.

Implementing a quality improvement process is essential to the long-term viability of the public health system, not least because it can achieve efficiencies. Quality improvement processes focus the staff on improving and streamlining the patient experience and often resources are saved as a result. One fewer mistake means one fewer mess to clean up. Around 20% of hospital spending goes on treating potentially preventable medical cock-ups.[196] This can't be cut overnight, but there are ways of reducing the cost over time. Spending increases are likely to be limited in coming years, so quality improvement could be vital to free up resources whilst also improving treatment quality.

Mistakes are a major source of inefficiency, but there are others. A striking thing that emerges in conversation with surgeons from up and down the country is how often they commented on the inefficiency present in public sector delivery of surgery. Theatres are taken at a moment's notice to deal with an emergency. Patients don't turn up. The pace of turnaround between operations is much slower – one surgeon commented that it normally took around half an hour between operations in the public sector, whereas it was five minutes in the private sector. Patients lounge around in beds in the public sector longer, too.

At the root of it all are incentive problems. They emanate from the top and impact on the whole health sector. DHBs get paid a slug of money – their only real performance criterion is not to overspend, and most of them fail at that. They face few incentives to worry about improved prevention, or about doing more and safer operations. This lack of incentive gets passed on to staff, who usually either face no incentives to improve performance, or face incentives to avoid safety problems. Surgeons told us that public sector administrators tended to view treatments as a cost – that is, something to be avoided – while the private sector viewed treatments as revenue, something to be encouraged. This might explain why the extra money put into the public sector in recent years has achieved so little. People have just kept doing what they have always done, with more money to spend.

Improving the way hospitals are run is a massive opportunity to improve our health and save money at the same time.[197] Health workers tend to be focused on caring for individual patients, so thinking about processes such as quality and efficiency is all a bit of an anathema. Little short of a cultural change is required.

Whai Manaaki – manufacturing meets medicine

Toyota became a global giant car maker through its principle of Kaizen – constantly improving quality, which both reduces mistakes and saves money. Counties Manukau, working with other DHBs, is applying these techniques in their hospitals. Will we see nurses in greasy overalls? Not really, but the principle is the same – reduce mistakes and distractions, and have more time to care for patients.

Involving staff is key to the whole process. Front line staff start by devising their own performance measures, which are reported publicly to show their progress. Then they identify and solve problems with the aim of improving on those measures. External coaches work with staff to shift the culture and introduce Toyota style tools to help solve their own problems. This takes longer but means that the change is permanent. Buy-in from the top of the hospital is also essential to kick-start changes.

There are many benefits to this approach. Most impressively, around 90% of all patients in emergency department are now treated or discharged within six hours – up from around 65% in 2008. Staff turnover is down too, as people feel more empowered to make changes in their roles.

Storerooms and inventories have been organised – improving access for staff and freeing up space for other uses. Mobile telephone handsets allow nurses to spend more time with patients and less answering calls from concerned families. Computerised drug dispensing has reduced mistakes (which previously occurred in up to a third of patients) and cut the amount of drugs that gets chucked away. The money saved paid back the investment in equipment within three months. One ward put in place an improved discharge process which not only frees up beds quicker, it also checks the patient's medication list for possibly dangerous drug 'cocktail' effects. Only 69% of patients in New Zealand have this check done when they leave hospital. This is surprising when it's such a simple and cost-effective way of reducing mistakes.[198]

As greater importance is being put on primary care, similar efficiency and quality issues are arising there. We've already mentioned that the future of dealing with chronic disease lies in the delivery of coordinated care by a team of primary care professionals, including GPs, nurses, physios, nutritionists and pharmacists. This sort of approach is much easier to deliver in larger, integrated clinics. It just so happens that these clinics also tend to be more efficient to run because of economies of scale, and because other professionals can do the things that GPs used to do. Nurses can easily do many of the required tasks – such as a routine health check-up. Just like provincial hospitals, the old-style local GP clinics are becoming an outdated mode of delivering primary care to the population.

Labour's primary healthcare reforms were intended to incentivise a move to larger, team-based primary practices, but perversely they may have had the opposite effect. In the past, GPs tended to cluster in affluent areas, as they depended on rich folks for their fee income. This means that affluent areas have high numbers of GP practices, each with few patients – a pretty inefficient model. Because Labour boosted funding without capping fees, these practices could significantly boost their incomes – which may have kept many of them running and prevented change. Labour's huge funding injection did not always lead to significantly lower GP fees, particularly in affluent areas. The result was that the average profit of a full-time practising GP *doubled* between 2001 and 2006 to $186,600.[199] Meanwhile, GPs were enjoying the new high life by reducing their hours – since 2000 they work on average 3.6 hours *less* per week (a 9% reduction). In poorer areas, Labour got the incentives right: new services are being delivered in large-scale, integrated clinics, which can afford to service the local populace with a limited fee income.[200] These clinics tend to employ GPs and nurses rather than having them run their own business, and for many young GPs, this is an attractive option. This is how Labour hit its fee reduction targets in poor areas, even if it failed in affluent ones.

So if improving efficiency in the primary sector relies on establishing more large-scale clinics, why haven't more been set up? The inertia for GPs is understandable. Setting up a team-based clinic – or 'super-clinic' as some refer to them – takes a lot of time and money. Many are nearing the end of their careers and don't want to change everything now. The recent funding boost has allowed them to delay change further. And many of the larger PHOs are unlikely to set up new super-clinics because it would put them in competition with established GP practices, who are their members, after all. If change is to come, it will need to be through outside intervention by DHBs and the Ministry of Health.

Summary

While we need professional administrators running our health sector, it's hard to argue with the frequently heard complaint that too much funding that could go into producing health outcomes is spent on central administration. The finger has been pointed at the Ministry of Health, when in fact the DHBs are the problem. There is too much fat in the DHB system, with unnecessary duplications and fragmentation. It's difficult to see a rationale for the present DHB system other than a political expedience, driven (or at least, conditioned) by a fear of parochial defensiveness about local hospitals. The level of services in smaller DHBs is poor and deteriorating, and meanwhile, an unacceptable level of cross-subsidisation threatens the viability of the larger DHBs, which are obliged to pick up the slack. The hospital services sector is long overdue for rationalisation.

Labour's heart was in the right place when it boosted funding and placed increased emphasis on the primary sector, but the efflorescence of PHOs was both unexpected and unhelpful. There are a range of PHOs, and they are either good at reaching their communities or at capturing economies of scale, seldom both. Some rationalisation of PHOs is necessary to fully realise the intention of the reforms.

Quality Improvement offers the win-win of improved health alongside leaner and meaner delivery. Administrators and medical staff will need to work together to achieve this. No part of the health sector should drown in unnecessary paperwork, nor should any part be above ongoing monitoring, improvement and evaluation. No doubt some will whinge, but good performers have nothing to fear, except maybe receiving some recognition for their work.

Chapter 9

CAN WE SAVE IT?

Before we go on to talk about the problems that the present health system suffers from and how they might be fixed, let's spend a little bit of time cutting it some slack. We do a lot of stuff well, and looking at our strengths can give us some clues on how best to address our weaknesses.

We're better off with our strange hybrid of funding models – a little bit of private, a little bit of social insurance, a lot of public – than a lot of nations that have a hell of a lot more money to throw at health than we do. America, for example, is having discussions about their health system right now that make the most heated debate in New Zealand look like a pleasant chat over tea and biscuits. In absolute terms, we run our healthcare system on the smell of an oily rag, and yet we're among the longest-lived and healthiest people in the world (ignoring, for the present, because we're being upbeat about this, exceptions to the rule such as Maori and Pacific Islanders). America, by contrast, is the world's undisputed heavyweight big spender on health, and its outcomes suck by comparison with ours, particularly for those at the bottom of the heap. Our own, mildly redistributive system focuses on need, and does a reasonable job of addressing it.

We tackle the thorny issue of prioritisation pretty well. We are commendably willing to put money into public health and preventive medicine, despite the 'rule of rescue' that says people prefer to spend cash on screaming, writhing, suffering victims of illness and accident than on the faceless masses who, suppose the money has been spent wisely, will never reach that stage. Our biggest success stories in this department have been our fight against smoking – we have one of the lowest rates of smoking and therefore smoking-related illness in the developed world – and our struggle with heart disease, where preventive measures and the use of effective drugs such as statins have made real, measurable improvements in the lives of New Zealanders over the last 30 years. It's all very well for politicians to bleat about waiting lists for hospital procedures, but doing so overlooks how sensible it has been to focus resources on the primary system, which is where prevention and early intervention – that stitch in time – take place.

Pharmac has been a resounding hit. You can prove this by comparing our national spend on pharmaceuticals with the rest of the world, but the real giveaway is how much the Americans hate it. It's a model of how research together with clear, settled principles can provide a pole star for decision-makers to steer by as they're tossed about in the murkiest reaches of the ethical deep.

Our emergency care is exemplary. Generally, if you find yourself with an acute, life-threatening condition, you stand as good a chance of pulling through as it's humanly possible to provide, thanks to the quality of the emergency care in our hospitals. And while we're counting our blessings, this points to one of the greatest blessings of all, the quality of our healthcare workers. Many of the present crop have lived through an era of immense upheaval, and to those who are still standing, we must be eternally grateful. Some staff feel they're undervalued by those who make decisions about and within the system: many of the experts to whom we spoke emphasise the importance of involving the system's skilled and dedicated workforce in any further changes that are proposed. The entire history of previous reforms underscores the importance of this point. Bring the staff along with you, and the reforms succeed. Try to drag them by the nose and you're doomed to fail.

Future challenges

As we have seen, despite our relatively good performance, there's no room for complacency. On the contrary: there are many healthcare challenges looming on the horizon. The ageing population is a big one, but surprisingly not the biggest. The major problem is going to be the increasing disparity between what we expect and what the system is going to be able to deliver. Experience shows that people simply expect more treatment for the same condition than they did in the past – and doctors want to provide it, too. The range of treatments available grows daily, and treatments are becoming more technologically intensive. We're competing in a global market for healthcare professionals, and they're a scare resource themselves. Healthcare costs are therefore always going to be on an upward trend. The recession of the last little while has spelt an end to the era of easy credit, so there seems no prospect of the government injecting ever more money in the fiscal equivalent of collagen injections, giving it that spurious, pink-of-health glow. We already ration our healthcare, and as resources become scarcer, the need to prioritise is going to be more acute.

Those making the prioritisation decisions are going to be juggling three balls: end-of-life, prevention (versus cure) and chronic disease.

Treatment at the end-of-life can be expensive, and could potentially become a greater expense, given our ageing population. Yet many last-ditch attempts to save someone's life are driven by the medical staff and the family for their own ends rather than out of genuine consideration for the patient. How mad is that? Medical professionals need to front up and honestly communicate the risks and downsides of treatment. Without this information we, the families, too often keep our loved ones alive past the point where there's any prospect of giving them quality of life, simply to assuage our guilt and to be sure we 'did everything we could'. We are long overdue a public conversation about the balance between end-of-life treatment and care, and how we can best manage people's final farewell from this existence. We are cracking out the defibrillator when the heart monitor flat-lines, when perhaps a caring caress will do. This will take a great deal of maturity from all concerned. Most of us (doctors included) don't feel that comfortable talking about death, especially not the death of loved ones. Elderly people can feel (understandably) threatened by the thought of a discussion taking place of when and under what circumstances their family will switch off the machine. Maybe it is better to start with what we value in life, so that our families can understand under what circumstances we don't want to be resuscitated. This would improve quality of life, and however distasteful it may seem, it will probably save money too. These conversations take place every day, too often when the useful time for them has passed. And with our greying population, this topic – along with pensions and retirement homes – will be increasingly hard to avoid over the next twenty years.

As we've just been discussing, prevention really is better than cure. Money spent on prevention or early intervention makes us healthier for longer than money spent on cures. This includes doing operations for 'minor' conditions before they become major ones. The only problem is that providing the cure is more visible to the media and public than prevention is. Again, this is an issue worthy of a public conversation. If we invest more in prevention, and live longer, healthier lives as a result, are we prepared to have less treatment available to us when our bodies finally pack in? Or, to paraphrase James Dean do we prefer to live fast, die young, and leave a heavily medicated corpse?

Chronic disease is not new, but the size of the future burden could be a real challenge. One problem that is looming large – no pun intended – is the soaring rate of obesity among New Zealanders. Obesity isn't a disease in itself, but it can be the cause and aggravating factor in a whole constellation of diseases and disorders and a complicating factor in surgery. Our health system isn't well suited to addressing these kinds of problem: it's much better at one-off, quick fixes. Dealing with increased rates of chronic disease will require changing the way health care is delivered – teams of primary carers will need to work in partnership with the patient to manage conditions and prevent those expensive hospital visits. This kind of change can't take place without considerable investment, and preferably in anticipation of the problem rather than waiting until our hand is forced.

Changes

If you do not change the direction in which you are going, you will end up where you are headed.

Confucius

Some of the experts we talked to outlined one Doomsday scenario wherein enough of the middle class became disenchanted with the public health system and switched to private insurance. This would change the political dynamics so voters would no longer demand an efficient, effective public healthcare system. In this vision the public sector would dwindle as the poor cousin and we'd all go private – except the poorest, of course. We'd end up like America.

At the moment, this seems pretty far-fetched. The public system isn't disappearing anytime soon. The private sector will no doubt expand as the public system confronts burgeoning demand, but let's not get too excited about the private sector taking over our healthcare system just yet.

While we don't want to go altogether private, however, one change that is urgently needed is to get the politicians out of as many aspects of the present system as we can. We need, that is, to depoliticise health. Our politicians show in everything they do – and their lily-livered attempts at reforming the health sector over the last three decades have been no exception – that they're hopelessly in the thrall of public opinion, no matter how ill-informed, misguided or deluded public opinion might happen to be. We don't need people calling the shots whose primary interest is in how readily their decision is going to convert to votes. The health sector has suffered too much from this kind of meddling through the years.

Treatment prioritisation

The greatest disappointment of the Labour years was the retreat from the debate on prioritisation. The case of poor old Rau Williams initially shocked New Zealanders, but we eventually started to have a reasonably mature discussion about where our healthcare budget should go. But politicians got spooked by the backlash. The National/NZ First coalition elected in 1996 started the retreat, and this run for cover was continued by Helen Clark's Labour-led Government in 1999. Soon we were all back in nanny state wonderland, with ailing DHBs kept open literally at any cost and the grand delusion of free, universal healthcare allowed to rule OK.

Admitting that prioritisation goes on is political suicide, but sooner or later the New Zealand public needs to be shown the equation so that our expectations can be recalibrated to match our resources. Then public debate will be needed over what our healthcare priorities really are.

It will be a brave politician who sets this ball rolling, particularly after the cropper the National Government of the 1990s came. But that government went out seeking a political consensus instead of trying to walk the public through an impartial, un-emotive basis for decision-making such as the QALY and CPAC systems. It takes time for people to understand the choices that need to be made, and any given politician only has three years to get anything done, even suppose they're willing to try. For this reason, politicians are the wrong people to communicate the ins and outs of prioritisation to the public. Their popularity is too precious to them to raise the hard questions and defend the framework in the face of a rabid, self-interested assault by the knobbly-kneed grey brigade. These messages would be far more powerful coming from doctors.

Perhaps a good place to start would be in explaining to the public just how Pharmac works. After all, it's seen overseas as international best practice in pharmaceutical purchasing. Sure, there are arguments, usually about the strength of evidence used in making decisions, but at least these arguments are all out in the open. No decision goes unscrutinised or untested, and at the root of every decision is a calculation based on the amount of QALYs – quality adjusted life years – that the proposed funding will achieve for patients receiving the subsidised drug. That's a vast improvement on what happens in the prioritisation of treatments at the moment, where decisions are at the mercy of a bunch of no-names meeting behind the closed doors of the DHB boardroom, or of the jerking knee of a Minister of Health every time s/he reads a newspaper headline signalling rumblings of discontent in the electorate.

For about two years, New Zealand had something called the Health Funding Authority (HFA), which was a version of Pharmac for medical treatments. It helped prioritise spending and was a move away from the much-maligned competitive model, but being a National Party creation it was an early target for scrapping when the Labour-led Government came to power. But most experts in the health system we interviewed felt it was the best system of treatment prioritisation New Zealand has ever had.

Making a Pharmac for medical treatments – or 'Sickmac' if

you will – fly wouldn't be easy. After all, it's not easy to come by the information that helps decision-makers put money where it gives the greatest health benefit. It takes time to gather, and would probably require information sharing with overseas institutions like the UK's National Institute for Health and Clinical Excellence (NICE), which is already some way down this road. But we could start by looking closely at the really important treatments, like heart disease, diabetes, strokes, cancer and respiratory illnesses. Best-practice prevention and treatments could be worked out, and a uniform set of standards of treatment (guidelines, quality measures, treatment thresholds, quantity of operations, acceptable waiting times, etc) applied across the country. Then we could see how that went and if it worked, extend the model. This would be a step toward defining core services, which we should have been able to do twenty years ago. There could still be local flexibility outside of these central services, but we'd all benefit from having the certainty this system provided.

STOP PRESS: The Horn Report

As this book went to print, the Government was preparing its response to a slew of reviews that have been done in its first year of power. The biggest of these – the 'Horn Report' – was prepared by a Working Group headed by Murray Horn, former Secretary to the Treasury. To banish fears of a return to the dog-eat-dog approach of the 1990s, National promised that there would be no reform of the DHB structure. Instead, they pledged to reduce bureaucrats in favour of more docs and nurses (presumably they won't just give the bureaucrats a scalpel). National may come to rue these promises, because the Horn Report struggles to accommodate them both.

The Horn Report sets out all the same problems we have seen in this book – a health system addicted to injections of cash, but still struggling to meet public expectations for treatment. It points to some similar solutions too, by signaling a return to national purchasing similar to the Health Funding Authority (HFA). National's new HFA (called a National Health Board) would only purchase a few specialised national procedures to start with.

Let's hope this role is successful and quickly expands to cover the really important health conditions, like cancer and heart disease. There is some attempt to have Pharmac-style prioritisation for medical treatments too through a National Health Committee. But instead of putting this group within the National Health Board so it had the power to spend money in the national interest as Pharmac does, it will merely report to the Minister. This wimpy structure will mean the Minister continues to get his sticky paws all over prioritisation decisions, and is unlikely to help much.

The Report proposes another central agency to purchase shared services on behalf of all DHBs. However, it was precluded from taking things to their logical conclusion – disbanding smaller DHBs and culling provincial hospitals. As a compromise, we keep all the DHBs but gain a couple of new central agencies. How exactly does this half-assed, halfway-house solution get us fewer bureaucrats? It is time to completely review the healthcare *services* we want as a country and then work out the best way of delivering them, rather than pandering to those who want to be on a Hospital Board, or have a hospital in their one-horse town.

The Horn Report chases the savings from investing in quality improvement and information technology. This should improve efficiency over time, despite further increases in central bureaucracy. These initiatives will hopefully join up with National's plans for staff to have more say in the running of hospitals. In fact, things look pretty rosy for medical staff: the Government is doing a lot to promote the training and retention of staff. Perhaps they are doing too much. If there are too many doctors, it stops innovation in the delivery of services.

In short, the Government has some important reforms on the table that could improve the functioning of the hospital sector, but it's allowing itself to be hamstrung by its own electioneering tactics. In order to exorcise the ghost of Nationals past, they promised not to do exactly what needs to be done – reform DHBs. They need either to set out a long term plan, or risk the reforms tripping over their own contradictions. They also need to recognise that these reforms alone will not be enough to prevent our health system buckling under future demands. The challenges are bigger than some tinkering in Wellington can solve. What's needed is nothing short of cultural change which accommodates the honesty of a clear and well-known definition of what is and what isn't within the ambit of the public health system.

A 'Sickmac' model would be a dramatic improvement on the current system. At the moment, priorities are governed by catastrophes. Under David Cunliffe, heart disease was the big panic. Now Tony Ryall is stressed about cancer treatment. Each administration makes big pronouncements about the inadequacy of treatments in certain areas and how the situation has to change. DHB boards kowtow to Ministers, and hurriedly rearrange resources to meet the new standards so that the Minister can claim success. Meanwhile another service falls over, ready to give the next Minister an opportunity to be the knight in shining armour. It all is quite distasteful when, meanwhile, there are New Zealanders being denied cost-effective treatments and others being provided expensive interventions with minimal benefit. It smacks more of political gaming than any rigorous appreciation of the health sector as a whole, and that's just criminal.

As we saw in Chapter Four, the QALY alone wouldn't be a sufficient criterion for this system, because it overlooks clinical suitability and the moral element of our decision-making (a consideration of the relative benefits of the same treatment to different patients). So a more subtle prioritisation framework would be needed, one that is based on the best QALY evidence available to medical staff and to informed citizens. There are a variety of models in use overseas that combine all three of these elements. Each has its merits, but the important point is that each benefits from including the three most vitally interested parties without allowing politicians to contaminate the rational decision-making process with rank populism.

Have your say

In 1997 the Southern and Midland Regional Health Authority both embarked on a 'Programme Budgeting and Marginal Analysis' known as PBMA.

These are some fancy words for getting docs, administrators and the public together to decide what things they should do more of and what they should do less of. The exercise looked at the evidence on treatment for respiratory diseases and reached similar conclusions in both regions. Smoking cessation was ranked the most important investment by both regions, and both regions agreed that further high priorities included community-based consultant clinics, sleep apnoea services, educating health professionals on respiratory issues and improving the quality of prescribing.[201]

As in the Herceptin debacle, lots of advocates for certain treatments or screening campaigns focus on the benefits without looking at the costs. A good example was the successful campaign to lower the minimum age for mammographic screening from 50 to 45 years. Use of a 'citizens' jury', a system that is already used widely in Sweden, was trialled to test this decision. The jury was drawn from a random sample of women. They were advised by a range of experts, some of whom opposed the change in eligibility, some of whom were in favour, and some of whom were neutral. Initially, the majority of the jury were in favour of the increased screening. After a day and a half hearing evidence and half a day of deliberation, however, the jury decided that on balance, the additional screening was not justified.[202] Not only does such screening come at a cost that outweighs the benefit, there is also the potential for harm from the screening process. Sadly, this hasn't changed national policy. Breast screening is still available from 45 years of age.

The greatest benefits of such an approach are that there's a framework that's not ad hoc and subject to corruption by political agendas, and it means the way our health budget is spent is out in the open for all to see, rather than based on opaque processes, personalities and the dead hand of history. This would give it more stability. The only question is: are we grown up enough to have the conversation that we need to have? Or will we crumple every time a special interest group gets on the telly à la Herceptin and corrupts the process?

Quality improvement
International evidence shows that the top performers in the healthcare world relentlessly track and transparently report their performance and back this up with appropriate incentives (this doesn't always mean money). This applies at all levels – from healthcare organisations right down to individual staff.[203] [204] Depending on your experience, this concept might sound blatantly obvious, but it's pretty alien to many working in our health system. Not surprisingly, though, simply having transparent reporting of the right measures can make a big difference to performance. Even without incentives to improve, at the very least people get shamed into upping their game, and they start learning off those who are doing better. Overseas experience shows that this is far more effective than the spurious fillip of business-style 'competition' between hospitals.

Should patients know how good their doctors are?[205]

Annie Page's dad used to call her Little Potato Chip, because her skin tasted salty when he kissed her. Annie was always small, and after a bunch of tests they realised she had cystic fibrosis. This is a genetic disease which clogs the lungs with mucus, slowing the body's growth and eventually causing premature death. But the disease is manageable, and life can be dramatically extended. But by how much?

Data has been collected on cystic fibrosis programmes across the USA for years, but it was only provided to the hospitals and even then with hospital names removed. The data was used by authorities to develop good practice guidelines and this alone had already led to dramatic improvements – the average life expectancy of a CF sufferer had risen from three years in 1957 to 33 years in 2003. But the best performers were always ahead of the pack, and by 2003 they were up to 47 years.

Four years after Annie's diagnosis, Annie's hospital decided to inform its patients what it knew about relative performance.

Their new head of medicine was convinced that the only way the hospital and the whole industry could improve was by measuring their performance and being up front and honest about it. Their results were not great – the hospital was average – and the doctors were nervous about how the patients would take it. Would they want to move elsewhere? Amazingly, none did. The patients and doctors sat down and worked out how they were going to get better.

Part of their improvement plan was to see how the top performers did it. This proved difficult to find out, because there is such resistance to openness in sharing healthcare performance data. Annie's parents kept pushing and eventually they did find out, and are continuing to campaign for more transparency and openness. In the end their concern was not so much whether their daughter's hospital was average – someone always has to be average – but whether they were doing anything about it. Continuous improvement is all anyone can ask.

The big problem is that the quality of reporting in our health sector is still pretty poor, yet this is an essential starting point for a more mature, depoliticised debate about healthcare in New Zealand. We don't have firm answers even to obvious questions, such as: what is the prevalence of conditions in different areas? What is the demand for treatment for different conditions (this may be different to prevalence, due to some conditions going undiagnosed)? What is the capacity to treat different conditions? What are waiting times for treatment and the levels of unmet need for different treatments? How much do different treatments cost to deliver in different regions? How effective are different treatments in different hospitals, or under different doctors? What is the chance that your treatment will go wrong in different hospitals, or with different doctors?

Partly, the gathering and reporting of such information is difficult because our health sector lacks decent information technology. Several senior administrators we talked to said they would love to make this sort of long-term investment, but in the current environment, couldn't divert sufficient resources from the short-term focus of treating people. Even where good IT systems exist, they can't be compared, let alone integrated across the sector, and getting a nationwide, integrated system would require the DHBs to work together. No one's managed that yet, and successive governments have failed to show leadership and push through a more coordinated approach.

Once the information has been gathered, it ought to be made available to interested parties, including the public who, after all, have the right to know whether their taxes are being spent wisely and effectively. Healthcare workers are unlikely to appreciate too much additional transparency. Ultimately, though, a good deal of maturity from the media, consumers, taxpayers and doctors alike will be needed to make this work. Some sort of requirement to gather and report information ought to have been imposed on DHBs in return for the cash injections and salary hikes made by the last Labour-led government. It looks like that was a huge missed opportunity.

Once we have the right kind of information, we can encourage continuous improvement against an agreed set of measures, backed by appropriate incentives. Measures and targets at the moment are quite piecemeal and generally not linked to incentives. Where they are set, they tend to be politically driven – the manipulation of waiting times and the merry-go-round of quixotic championing by Health Ministers of the treatment of one group of diseases at the expense of others are prime examples. Ill-considered targets can cause some absurd distortions. In the UK, for example, when there was a target to reduce waiting times in A&E, some hospitals kept people in ambulances out in the reception bay and only admitted them when they were ready to treat them. But well-designed targets and incentives have been shown to improve health sector performance, too.[206] A good example (again from the UK) was an incentive offered to GPs to reduce smoking and increase vaccination rates among their patients. We could even go further. Everyone could have regular medicals (with the frequency depending on age) and over time primary care providers could be rewarded for their ability to manage issues like weight, blood sugar, blood pressure and cholesterol amongst their patients. For chronic patients, reducing hospitalisation rates could be rewarded. Clearly measures, targets and incentives need to be used sparingly and to be focused on areas where there is strong evidence that it will make a difference. Any targets set also need to be sensitive to the starting point, and so achievable. Otherwise their relevance is never accepted.

Once the information is available to determine what's going right and wrong in the health sector – including what the effect of targets and incentives has been – evaluation can close the loop, and the information be used to set new targets and incentives.

The incentives used to improve quality can range from pride to monetary reward. For treatments outside those identified as core, there could be more widespread experimentation with the way health providers are funded. Imagine bulk-funding a hospital unit and telling staff that any savings they make will be open for reinvesting in their unit if there's a surplus. They would finally have an incentive to get engaged in innovating and improving the operation of the unit, to work with GPs on prevention (to reduce the number of patients admitted to their unit) and to avoid over-treating patients – the supplier-induced demand problems that have kept cropping up, like the proverbial bad penny, throughout this book.

The reform of the primary health sector aimed to create incentives for GPs to focus on preventing health problems. In truth these incentives never fully materialised. Partly, this was because GPs still charge a co-payment for each visit a patient makes, and partly it's because their responsibilities were never clearly defined. When a patient becomes too ill, for example, a GP can simply pack them off to hospital. The role of the hospital as back-up dilutes the GP's responsibility. More explicitly defined incentives could encourage them to focus on preventive health issues. As mentioned, imagine if GPs were rewarded for successfully managing their patient's smoking, immunisation and weight issues. We could also pay fees to GPs with a 'special interest' for each procedure they undertook which might prevent serious future conditions, like removing moles. GPs could even assume responsibility for managing pharmaceutical and diagnostic budgets. After all, they currently make spending decisions in these areas but don't face any incentives to manage costs.

Cellulitis Waikato[207]

The rule of rescue often means that our healthcare system treats the urgent instead of the important. The focus on life saving treatments means that simple procedures don't get done which save money in the long term. One example of the impact of treating small conditions early is cellulitis (basically a spreading skin infection). Acute cellulitis can be treated by GPs with a simple procedure costing around $250, however most GPs are not funded for this activity. If it goes untreated it can result in a visit to the emergency department with a price tag of $3,700.[208]

Waikato DHB has worked with its GPs to ensure they all have the same treatment and management approach for cellulitis in adults. Less than 9% of the 1300 adults treated for cellulitis in primary care require referral to emergency departments. The rate of avoidable hospitalisation for cellulitis in Waikato DHB is 75–90% of the national average.

It's likely that public funding of healthcare will hit a wall over the next few years, and part-charges for hospital treatment are an obvious response. Charging for GP care and not hospital care is frankly bizarre in terms of the evidence of benefit to society and our lifespan. Some payment could be sought for hospital care from those who can afford it, particularly for non-urgent care. Payments could potentially increase as a proportion of the total cost depending on the level of patient need or the priority of the operation type. This funding could be used to reduce the cost of GP visits, increase public sector surgical procedures, as well as to increase the amount of minor procedures done in primary care.

Capital

DHBs are pretty effective at making large investments in their own area, but very poor at doing anything that requires working together. It's not recommended that anyone hold their breath waiting for the 21 DHBs to collaborate in establishing a nationally integrated IT system, for example. National committees like NSTR (see Chapter Two) need to be given a budget to back up their decisions, because they're never going to tear DHBs away from parochial interests long enough to get them to focus on the national good.

The process for making decisions about large capital investments is laborious enough under the present system, then, without the interference of pork-barrelling politicians, who like to have a shiny new building to open every now and again, particularly in a marginal electorate. After all, everyone likes to see a new hospital (or unit) open; no one likes to see one close.

Given how hard the decisions are, and how fraught they become when politicians are involved, we need to remove long-term investment decisions from the clammy hands of Ministers. A buffer insulating decision makers from public opinion might even allow tough decisions – such as the closure of small, unviable hospitals – to be made and resources thus to be freed up for more productive investment in other areas.

Numbers of administrators and DHBs

The current, burgeoning number of administrators is an expression of our parochial health system, and of the deluded notion that there can be a fully equipped and functioning hospital

on every provincial street corner. The spread of hospitals and of
services is long overdue for rationalisation. Some thought needs
to be given to what key services we want provided across the
nation, what is the minimum size of hospital needed to deliver
those services, and where those services should be based.
The bad news is that if this is done right, some hospitals and
some units within existing hospitals would be merged or shut
down. Either that, or provincial hospitals will be dependent on
local charity to keep them afloat, which is not beyond the bounds
of possibility in the future. How many small towns have regular
fundraisers for their volunteer fire brigade?

So how many DHBs do we need? This question is really
a red herring. The real question is at what geographic level
should different services be provided? Once that is resolved, the
appropriate administration and local accountability structures
will follow.

Evidence from Ireland[209] suggests that the *minimum* population
needed for an effective accident and emergency unit is 200,000-
250,000. The full range of regional services requires 300,000-
350,000. 'Supra-regional' specialities require 750,000-1,000,000
people, whereas national services are, well, national.

Applying this methodology to the smallest DHBs means
we would probably need roughly 12 A&E units. New Zealand
currently has 35. Sure, we are a spread out country and some
analysis would need to be done to make sure that travel times
in an emergency weren't too long. But travel times can't justify
having three times the number of A&E units – if the population
analysis is correct, either we must close a few hospitals, or you
folks in the West Coast and Wairarapa need to get breeding.

But suppose we shut down Greymouth's hospital? What would
Coasters do for emergency treatment? Like many remote areas of
New Zealand, they would need to rely on a flying doctor service,
and the good news is that small regional airlines tend to have

flight reliability of 95-98%.[210] Indeed, according to pilots, it's not Greymouth that has to worry about weather disruption: Wanaka is far trickier to fly into, but luckily all the ski bunnies can hop in their 4WD SUVs to get treatment if they have to.

On a more serious note, the void left by the closure of unviable provincial hospitals would likely be filled by more sophisticated primary care, especially since the funding that had previously been slung down the gurgler at the hospital would be available to give them a boost. Primary super-clinics could perform minor operations (quality assured by clinical networks) and have some beds so that people can recover from surgery closer to home.

So what services should be supplied at each level? This would need to be worked through in some detail, but some examples are obvious. Paediatric oncology is a good one. Wellington's paediatric oncology service has been unstaffed four times in the past ten years, and it has made the headlines on each occasion. In April 2009, the latest two staff resigned after just five months in the job, forcing families with children under treatment there to travel to Christchurch or Auckland. The small scale of the unit makes it incredibly vulnerable to such problems. It serves around 500,000 people – too few for such a specialist service. Either the region covered by the unit needs to be increased, or it should cease operations entirely. But why would more people from outside Wellington want to use the service when there is already a superior service in Auckland?[211] Neurosurgery and plastic surgery are other examples of possible national units. Services like information technology, coordinating recruitment and training, capital spending plans and using evidence to develop treatment guidelines should also all be national. Complex surgery, like cardiac, should be done regionally, while minor surgery and emergency care needs to be based around cities of sufficient scale. Local services could be a boosted primary service that monitors and manages health risk factors (smoking, weight, diet, blood pressure, cholesterol, blood sugar levels), and conducts minor surgery.

This proposal will no doubt cause such uproar in some marginal electorates that no politician would contemplate it. However, the alternative is worse. Auckland will be the site of most of our population growth in coming years, and if it is shackled with bankrolling provincial hospitals (as it presently is), it will not be able to meet its own health needs. Meanwhile provincial hospitals will struggle along offering patchy service coverage. Everyone loses in this scenario. Having fewer, better hospitals would improve care and save money. The money freed up would allow the nation to make long-term investments, such as in world-class information technology to improve the coordination of the healthcare system. IT could also help overcome the tyranny of distance through e-consultations and telemedicine. Without such bold action, our health services face a long, slow decline of the kind we are starting to see now.

Health workers prefer working in environments with the facilities they need. They also respond to working in bigger teams, where it is possible to bond with and learn off other staff. For these reasons, most healthcare staff we talked to agreed that many hospital units and GP clinics could benefit from 'scaling up'. Any changes would need to make sure that the health system offered services as locally as possible, but with the scale required to offer an efficient and quality service. No medical staff would be out of work – we need all we can get. Some administrators would almost certainly find themselves surplus to requirement, as many of the roles that are duplicated poorly in 21 DHBs would be centralised.

What would we really lose by pruning the 21 DHBs and 80+ PHOs? It would hardly be a blow to democracy. Right now, local accountability really just means keeping the local hospital open. If we had decent monitoring data then any community group – such as local iwi – could hold the health system to account without the need to elect a Board. Thankfully, some of the sharper DHBs can see the writing on the wall – Otago and Southland are discussing a possible merger.

Should we spend more?

And now for the $12 billion question: should we spend more on our healthcare system? The answer depends on what you want from your health system. If you want gold-plated healthcare that guarantees you the latest treatments of a certain quality within a certain time and is tailored to you as an individual, then clearly we don't spend enough. We all need to get out our chequebooks and hand over another few cents out of every dollar we earn either to the government or to insurance companies. But European countries spend another 2-3 cents out of every dollar for this sort of care, and they too are now facing increasing bills given the ageing population – and don't forget they're already a damn sight richer than us. If, instead, we want a system that focuses on providing the most cost-effective treatments, gets the simple stuff right and can crank through high volumes of patients in a pretty uniform, standardised fashion, then we spend plenty already. We just need to focus less on the bleating of interest groups (doctors and patients alike) and deliver basic, evidence-based treatments with a focus on prevention and early intervention.

The reason we have fewer doctors and operations than many countries is because we are poorer. We can't afford to spend much more, and we probably can't even afford the current spending increases. Besides, if other countries are anything to go by, it's not clear that spending more on healthcare will create many benefits in terms of longer lifespan. Most modern healthcare systems are in diminishing marginal returns territory. As we get richer, we all want more and more treatment, and the docs are only too happy to oblige – hell, they even encourage it, because they love trying out the latest techniques, and besides, it all helps pay off the second Audi. But aside from placebo effects and having someone to hold our hand and tell us we will be okay, a lot of this extra care probably makes little difference to our health.

If we really want to live longer, it seems that quitting smoking, eating better and exercising more are just as likely to grant us those precious extra years of life as another visit to the operating table. Amazing as it seems, we might be just as well off making improvements in our lifestyle as we would be doubling healthcare spending, and lifestyle changes are clearly the cheaper option.

The heathcare system of the future

As we've seen, the New Zealand public healthcare system of the future will be very different from the one we're accustomed to today, partly because it will be shaped by different pressures – more of us presenting, most of us with the diseases of old age, many of us with chronic illness, particularly related to obesity – and partly, we hope, because we'll have learned by the mistakes of the past.

Kaiser Permanente[212]

This US health management organisation started out as part of a welfare system for factory workers like those provided by rich industrialists in Victorian times and the early 20th century. As the factories and shipyards shut down, Kaiser Permanente became a private insurance company with its own complete network of clinics and hospitals. Kaiser now has 8.6 million members, mostly in California. The doctors are salaried, but are shareholders and unlike the NZ public sector they cannot moonlight outside the Kaiser system.

Research indicates that Kaiser costs about the same to run as the UK's NHS system but generates better results, including lower waiting times and only one third of the rate of emergency admissions. Kaiser seems to achieve this through a heavy focus on prevention through promoting a healthy lifestyle, and having an integrated system where GPs and hospitals work closely together. Integration and coordination between providers is aided by a huge investment in information technology.

Kaiser saves money because it has lower rates of hospital admissions, and those people in hospital stay a shorter length of time. This hugely reduces costs without reducing the quality of care, and allows Kaiser to invest more funds in both prevention and information technology. Comprehensive, individual patient records allow Kaiser to spot potential negative trends and intervene early to help people prevent and manage any health problems before they require hospitalisation. High-risk patients are identified automatically by the information system and appointed a case manager to make sure they don't end up in hospital. So if your blood pressure suddenly shoots up you get a personal visit to make sure you are okay! The information the system provides also allows Kaiser to easily monitor what works and continuously improve its processes. Where the best practice evidence is clear, this is embedded in IT based guidelines for the treatment of certain conditions.

The backbone of this approach is Kaiser's paperless information technology system, which they invest 2% of their total health budget in maintaining and improving each year. Members can communicate with doctors, make and change appointments and view their patient record online.

The successes of the past should inform the reformers of the future. We have done brilliantly by international standards in reducing the rates of smoking and heart disease through the use of legislation, taxation, concerted public health campaigns and by addressing problems at the level of primary care. That, surely, has to point the way forward when it comes to tackling the next big public health issue, namely obesity. We've been slow out of the blocks on this one. When will we experience the equivalent of the epiphany that our society had about smoking and realise that obesity is becoming a crisis of similar proportions to the public health emergency that smoking became in the late 1960s? Probably when it is too late – by then schools will have replaced the TB jab with a diabetes test, and walking down the street will be like driving the dodgems. And yet, as a society, we have taken no action because of our concern over being a nanny state.

It's fine to stand on this principle so long as the 'nanny state' doesn't have to nurse the obese when they can no longer get out of bed. We either need to find a way of changing behaviour or start making life hard for those who live unhealthy lives, perhaps even by restricting entry to the health system. Getting serious about changing behaviour will mean taxing bad foods or subsidising good food, regulating advertising and labelling, mounting media campaigns with budgets to match McDonald's and even changing the layout of our cities – currently the car dominates, and walking and cycling are unattractive options. When will chocolate bars, fizzy drinks and chips carry large warnings of the clogged arteries and gangrene you risk developing, as a consequence of diabetes, from over-indulging in them? Restricting entry, on the other hand raises some tough moral issues – unless we simply put narrower doors on our hospitals and hope the fatties can't get in.

Public health or private profit?

In another of their bold reforms, the National Government of the 1990s set up a Public Health Commission – an independent body to advise the Government and invest in public health. The idea was brilliant – finally someone to focus on these big picture health issues. Sadly in practice the Commission was stymied from the outset. The split of responsibilities with the Ministry was not clear, leading to infighting, and the nail in the coffin was when the Commission angered the powerful tobacco, food and alcohol lobbies. They tried to stimulate a public conversation on how we should deal with issues like obesity and changes in our diet and exercise patterns, but were quickly silenced. What else were they supposed to do I wonder? This all proved too much for the National Government and it was buried after 18 months. This is a debate that urgently needs resurrecting.

Since the key to keeping everyone healthy on a budget lies in prevention, we need to think as laterally as we can about what constitutes holistic healthcare. It could be that the line between the health system and social welfare becomes blurred, or at least a little bit fuzzy. Encouraging a strong bond between mother and child has been shown to improve physical and mental health outcomes for both. Warm, dry housing helps in the fight against respiratory disease. Educating people about nutrition (or even taxing bad food) could help head off the obesity epidemic. Offering a helping hand during difficult times can prevent people going off the deep end. Where do you draw the line in what you spend your health dollar on?

After prevention, the next priority should be primary care, where we can probably expect to see a different model of general practice evolving. Most of our health costs are caused by a few people, who often have multiple health issues at the same time, including mental health. Case managers will work intensively with these people to steer them through the maze of treatment options available, and prevent problems before they happen. In some areas, there have already been steps taken toward developing the kind of partnership between primary care providers – doctors, nurses, pharmacists, physios, and so on – that we're going to need. These so-called 'super-clinics' will be where the hard yards are done in caring for the health needs of New Zealanders in the near future. By then, with luck (or good management – it's going to take one or the other), we'll have IT systems that facilitate the coordination of care in the primary system with whatever may be needed in the way of hospital treatment. GPs will work in partnerships, that is, rather than in silos.

And while we're on the subject of partnerships, the partnership between health workers and patients will become the most important relationship in the entire system. Some more than others, we urgently need to assume more responsibility for our health. And it could be that some of the work of managing illness, treatment and recovery is done by the 'expert patient' themselves, perhaps with the assistance of peer mentors.

One-stop (health) shop – Otaki Medical Centre

Carol moved around a bit when she was younger, but finally returned to her birthplace of Otaki on the Kapiti Coast around 30 years ago. Ever since then the Otaki Medical Centre has been her local GP. Six years ago Carol had a stroke, which left her in a wheelchair. At the time the Otaki Medical Centre was struggling along with two GPs. They got paid for each patient that visited them and the locals couldn't afford to pay much in terms of fees. So Carol's GP John Sprunt wasn't able to spend as much time as he would like with his patients – for example on preventing Carol's stroke, or helping rehabilitate her afterwards. Carol had to trek all the way to the hospital in Levin or Palmerston North for rehabilitation from her stroke.

Over time things have changed in the Otaki Medical Centre. They now get paid for each patient enrolled (rather than each visit), and they get more funding for patients that have high needs. John and his partner saw an opportunity to make the Centre sustainable and focus more on prevention. The Otaki Community Health Trust enlisted Dawn Wilson to help get the community behind this idea. They now have five GPs (plus one working part time) and six practice nurses, including one that works out in the community.

The local DHB has also based a further nine services in the Centre, with nurses and other health professionals providing expertise on managing heart disease, cancer, diabetes, respiratory problems, mental health issues, smoking, diet, exercise, and pharmaceuticals. Not only is the practice larger, it is more financially stable and the team atmosphere ensures there are fewer problems recruiting staff. Recruitment was a massive issue in the past – no Kiwi GPs have worked at Otaki for forty years. Almost everyone in the town is enrolled at the Centre – they have one of the highest enrolment rates in the country.

Carol has seen the practice grow over time, and it has made a big difference to the services she receives. Two years after her stroke a mental health nurse named Pam started at the centre. Pam became Carol's de facto case manager and helped her deal with her stroke and get the support she was entitled to.

Since then Carol was diagnosed with diabetes, and now she receives several regular services from the centre including regular blood tests, advice and encouragement on her diet and exercise regime.

All this support has prevented any further hospitalisation, and she no longer needs to trek up the road to Levin for treatment. The nurses have the time to help Carol change her lifestyle to ensure the problems don't recur. Most importantly everyone helping Carol is part of a team –they all share information on how she is doing through IT and meetings. Together they join up many different Government funding streams to look like a coherent package of services.

How times have changed. Now the citizens of Levin look with envy at the care Carol gets in Otaki. Horowhenua PHO has a number of solo GP operators, and none have managed to take the plunge to set up a large clinic like John Sprunt and his partner did. All across Horowhenua there are GP shortages. Dawn Wilson helps administer both PHOs and she puts the difference down to the Otaki Centre – a large clinic like Otaki is more appealing for doctors and offers a better service to patients too. As a result there are 40% more GPs per person enrolled in Otaki than there are in the Horowhenua PHO.

Thanks to the Otaki Medical Centre and particularly Pam's help, Carol's future is looking bright. Pam made sure that Carol was getting the help she needed to keep her independent in her own home. Carol has also wanted to give something back to the community for all the help she has received since her stroke, so Pam helped organise for Carol to qualify as an adult literacy tutor. Local people with literacy problems will soon be able to come to Carol's home for one-to-one help with their reading and writing problems.

Certainly, an emphasis on individual responsibility in health matters is part of the answer to the poor outcomes we currently see in Maori and Pacific Island communities. Community leaders need to encourage their members to foreswear their risky behaviours just as urgently as decision-makers in the health sector need to ensure that there are no barriers to access – whether it be financial, cultural, or even out-and-out racism – for any New Zealander. This will take reaching out to some communities.

Reaching out – Capital PHO

To the untrained eye, Wellington is a healthy place. The cafés are packed with earnestly health-conscious civil servants and Weta Digital techies, all ordering skim-milk, decaf lattes and munching on organic bran muffins. But beneath the surface Wellington has the same health problems as anywhere, particularly among Maori and Pacific Island communities. In some ways, all the affluence makes it harder to reach these communities, because the local GPs are used to dealing with the office gentry and can find it difficult to relate to other cultures.

Tui and Emma are the outreach nurses for the Maori and Pacific Island communities respectively in Wellington. They work for Capital PHO and aim to improve access to the health system for the 19,000 high-risk people in their area. Last year, Tui, Emma and their colleagues dealt with just under 500 referrals, reaching out to people who have fallen through the cracks of the health system. Most referrals come from GPs and are usually patients who need extra attention, or who have dropped off the radar. Tui and Emma make contact, explain they are from the GP, and generally get a warm reception – most people like and trust their 'Palagi GP'. They are only supposed to deal with the referral issue (e.g. vaccination), but often they find the health issues are far more complex, commonly involving an entire family.

Tui and Emma know that health sector funding can change as often as Tony Ryall's ties, and they may not still be there tomorrow. They focus on helping people to take charge of their own health. This might be through changing their diet, understanding hygiene, teaching them to communicate effectively with their doctor, how to budget so they can afford a smear test, or even discussing contraception. Some of the social issues they find are outside their role, so they have to maintain good networks and often end up referring families to a variety of healthcare and social services.

So far it seems to be working. They are seeing the right people – their patients are mostly poor and have high needs. More high-needs people are registered with their doctor in Wellington now than when the programme started.

If patience is a virtue, then Tui and Emma are saints. They meet people who don't do the simple things to keep themselves alive and healthy, and they often have to coordinate health services that don't talk to each other, even in the same hospital.

Some patients have to see more than one specialist. If they have diabetes, for instance, they are likely to have circulation or sight problems, too. Some patients assume that if they get held up seeing the ophthalmologist, that the cardiologist will know about it automatically and shift their appointment. Fat chance. Instead, when they turn up to the cardiologist, they are told that they missed their appointment and have to go to the back of the queue for another one. Often that can mean another six-month wait.

When things like this go wrong, some people bang the table and demand better service. Maori and Pacific Islanders tend to get embarrassed, stop listening and don't come back. No wonder they get fewer operations. The mainstream system can meet the health needs of these communities, but it will take a sustained effort from the likes of Tui and Emma and the people who had the vision to employ them to help the system improve – in particular getting Maori and Pacific Island communities understanding how to get the care they need. Some days it seems like an uphill battle, but they maintain their sanity by focusing on doing at least one positive thing for each family they see.

It's hard to imagine the public health system will get very far without a major rationalisation of services across the country. Some of the smaller hospitals will necessarily close, unless the population in their catchment grows spectacularly in numbers or in wealth. New models that remove the wasteful duplications in the current DHB system will need to be introduced, to streamline and coordinate funding and services.

A nationwide system of information-gathering and reporting will need to be developed, so that the government and the taxpayer alike can assess the value they're getting for their money. Improved monitoring will support continuous improvements in the health sector, which will lead to better quality services and reduced costs overall. And part of this will likely be the introduction of performance monitoring of healthcare workers, and the creation of incentives and targets. More public information on treatment risks might even ease the inexhaustible demand for operations.

We need to keep training healthcare professionals, and while it's unlikely we can prevent them availing themselves of market opportunities offshore, we need to ensure that our system is as good as any they can work in elsewhere in the world. Few enter these professions purely for the filthy lucre: if we can provide an efficient and effective environment in which they can apply their skills and feel they're doing their bit, we'll not only hang onto a good proportion of those we train locally, but we'll also become an attractive destination for the best and brightest of foreign-trained staff. This will require administrators to provide an environment where medical staff can focus on what they do best.

And whatever we do with the health system over the next crucial few years, we must make sure that the changes are made with the involvement and support of our health sector workers, who are, after all, the system's greatest asset and its most precious resource. We must not repeat the mistakes of the past.

Meanwhile, the rest of us need to talk. We need to discuss prioritisation – first to acknowledge the fact that it's unavoidable, and then to decide where we want to draw our lines. We'll need to inform ourselves about the relative merits of preventive medicine, primary care, and hospital services. And we'll need to give some thought to the criteria that are used to guide decisions both across treatments and within them – what treatments are funded, in other words, and who receives them. And given the inexorable trajectory of our demographics, a burning issue is going to be the decision to move our parents from end-of-life treatment to end-of-life care. This may mean spending a bit more on caring, so we can spend less on treatment at the end of life. Doctors and families alike will need to get real about how long modern healthcare can keep people alive and what it does to quality of life. CPR may work 70% of the time on the telly but the odds are only 25% in real life, and even then you may be nothing more than a glorified paperweight.

'Look to your health,' as the author of The Compleat Angler enjoined us. Look to it, indeed.

ENDNO✛ES

Introduction and Chapter 1

[1] Unless otherwise stated, all references in this Chapter are from Gauld, R. (2001) *Revolving Doors: New Zealand's Health Reforms*. Institute of Policy Studies and Health Services Research Centre

[2] New Zealand Historical Atlas, David Bateman, Auckland, 1997, panels 51, 55.

[3] http://www.eastonbh.ac.nz/?p=35

[4] 'Liabilities could sink ACC', Dominion Post, 9/10/09

[5] Source: North and South Magazine June 2005

[6] http://www.equity-for-illness.org.nz/case_studies.asp

[7] http://www.equity-for-illness.org.nz/case_studies.asp

[8] http://www.beehive.govt.nz/speech/speech+opening+counties-manukau+renal+dialysis+unit

[9] Manning, J and Paterson R (2005) *"Prioritisation" Rationing Health Care in New Zealand*, Legislating and Litigating Health Care Rights Around the World, Winter 2005 Issue

[10] http://www.eastonbh.ac.nz/?p=393

[11] Reported in Gauld, 2001

Chapter 2

[12] OECD Health Data

[13] Medical Council of New Zealand, The New Zealand Medical Workforce in 2008

[14] OECD (2007) *Health at a Glance 2007*

[15] SMO Commission (2009) *Senior Doctors in New Zealand: Securing the Future*

[16] World Health Organisation (2008) *World Health Statistics 2008*, WHO France

[17] OECD (2007) *Health at a Glance 2007*

[18] Ministry of Health (2008) *Briefing for the Incoming Minister of Health*

[19] All data from OECD Health Data 2008 unless otherwise stated.

[20] Ministry of Health and Minister of Health (2008) *Health and Independence Report 2008*. Wellington: Ministry of Health

[21] Ministry of Health (2008), *Briefing for the Incoming Minister of Health*

[22] Davis, P., Lay-Yee, R., Scott, A., & Gauld, R. (2007). Do hospital bed reduction and multiple system reform affect patient mortality? *A trend and multilevel analysis in New Zealand over the period 1988-2001. Medical Care*, 45, 1186-1194.

[23] Peter Davis, et al, (2002) *Adverse events in New Zealand public hospitals I: occurrence and impact*, Journal of the New Zealand Medical Association, 13-December-2002, Vol 115 No 1167

[24] Raymont, A., Hospital discharges in New Zealand 1991-2005: changes over time and variation between districts. New Zealand Medical Journal, 2008. 121(1279)

[25] http://www.statistics.gov.uk/cci/article.asp?ID=1922

[26] Ministry of Health and Minister of Health (2008) *Health and Independence Report 2008*. Wellington: Ministry of Health

[27] Lopez-Casanovas et al (2005) *Health and Economic Growth*, MIT

[28] http://en.wikipedia.org/wiki/Placebo

[29] Roberts & Kewman (1993) *The Power of Nonspecific Healing: Implications for Psychosocial and Biological Treatments* Clinical Psychology Review Vol 13, pp375-391

[30] Le Fanu, J *The Rise and Fall of Modern Medicine*, 1999

Chapter 3

[31] Le Fanu op. cit.

[32] Le Fanu op. cit.

[33] Joumard, I *et al* (2008) *Health Status Determinants – Lifestyle, Environment, Health Care Resources and Efficiency*, OECD Economics Department Working Papers No 627, OECD publishing

[34] Kjellstrand, CM, Kovithavongs, C & Szabo, E *On the Success, cost and efficiency of modern medicine: an international comparison*, Journal of Internal Medicine, 1998

[35] http://www.otago.ac.nz/news/news/2007/22-08-07_press_release.html

[36] Tobias, M et al (2009) *Changing trends in indigenous inequalities in mortality: lessons from New Zealand* Int J Epidemiol 2009 Mar 30

[37] www.facethefacts.org.nz

[38] www.facethefacts.org.nz

[39] Ministry of Social Development, (2008) *The Social Report*

[40] Tengs et al *Five Hundred Life-Saving Interventions and their Cost-Effectiveness*, Risk Analysis vol.15, No.3 1995

[41] MOH, Portrait of Health

[42] Average heights from OECD Society at a Glance 2009

[43] Ministry of Health (2008) *A Portrait of Health. Key Results of the 2006/07 New Zealand Health Survey.* Wellington: Ministry of Health

[44] World Health Organisation (2000) *The World Health Report 2000: Health Systems: Improving Performance* Switzerland WHO

[45] Ministry of Health (2008) *A Portrait of Health. Key Results of the 2006/07 New Zealand Health Survey.* Wellington: Ministry of Health

[46] Le Fanu, *The Rise and Fall of Modern Medicine*, Carroll & Graf, 1999

[47] Campbell, T.C. (2005) *The China Study*, Benbella Books, USA

[48] http://www.doctoryourself.com/laws.html

[49] Pollan, M (2008) *In Defence of Food*, Penguin (USA)

[50] Statistics are sourced from OECD Health Data 2008

[51] Ministry of Health and Minister of Health (2008) *Health and Independence Report 2008.* Wellington: Ministry of Health

[52] Ministry of Health (2008) *A Portrait of Health. Key Results of the 2006/07 New Zealand Health Survey.* Wellington: Ministry of Health

[53] Tobias, et al (2009) *Changing trends in indigenous inequalities in mortality: lessons from New Zealand* International Journal of Epidemiology 2009 1-12

[54] http://www.sciencedirect.com/science?_ob=ArticleURL&_udi=B6VBF-3X82T22-3&_user=10&_rdoc=1&_fmt=&_orig=search&_sort=d&view=c&_acct=C000050221&_version=1&_urlVersion=0&_userid=10&md5=93feadd64420a1cf8a4644d94d774a8e

[55] Subramanian & Kawachi (2004) *Income Inequality and Health: What Have We Learned So Far?* Epidemiol Rev 2004; 26:78-91

[56] Cohen & Henderson (1988) *Health, Prevention and Economics* Oxford OUP

[57] http://scotlandonsunday.scotsman.com/unemployment/Deadly-cost-of-unemployment.3691487.jp

[58] Gerdtham & Ruhm (2002) *Deaths Rise in Good Economic Times: Evidence From the OECD* IZA Discussion Papers 654, Institute for the Study of Labor (IZA)

[59] House et al, (1988) *Social Relationships and Health Science*, Vol 241, Issue 4865, 540-545

[60] Wilkinson, R. G., & Pickett, K. E. (2006). Income inequality and population health: A review and explanation of the evidence. *Social Science & Medicine*, 62(7), 1768-1784

[61] NZ Treasury (2001) *Tax Review 2001* Treasury, Wellington

[62] Most of this data is taken from the OECD Health Data 2008, although relates to the 2004 year.

[63] http://www.nzhis.govt.nz/moh.nsf/pagesns/528

[64] http://www.nzherald.co.nz/public-healthcare/news/article.cfm?c_id=294&objectid=10488362

[65] Ministry of Health (2008) *A Portrait of Health. Key Results of the 2006/07 New Zealand Health Survey.* Wellington: Ministry of Health

[66] Ministry of Health (2008) *A Portrait of Health. Key Results of the 2006/07 New Zealand Health Survey.* Wellington: Ministry of Health

[67] http://www.nzhis.govt.nz/moh.nsf/pagesns/528

[68] WHO website

[69] http://www.socialreport.msd.govt.nz/health/health-expectancy.html

[70] Barsky, A (1988) *The Paradox of Health*, New England Journal of Medicine

[71] Kroenke, K (1989) *Common Symptoms in Ambulatory Care: Incidence, Evaluation, Therapy and Outcome*, The American Journal of Medicine

[72] OECD (2007) *Health at a Glance 2007*

[73] Bunker, J *The Role of Medical Care*, International Journal of Epidemiology

[74] Tobias, M et al (2009) *Changing trends in indigenous inequalities in mortality: lessons from New Zealand* Int J Epidemiol 2009 Mar 30

[75] Statistics NZ March 2009 HLFS

[76] Source: Department of Labour (2009), *Labour Market Update*, May 2009

[77] Sporle A, Pearce N, Davis P. Social class mortality differences in Maori and non-Maori men aged 15–64 during the last two decades. N Z Med J. 2002; 115: 127–131.

[78] Ministry of Health (2008) *A Portrait of Health. Key Results of the 2006/07 New Zealand Health Survey*. Wellington: Ministry of Health

[79] Tobias M, Yeh L-C. How much does health care contribute to health gain and to health inequality? Trends in amenable mortality in New Zealand 1981-2004. Aust NZ J Public Health 2009; 33: 70-78

[80] Ministry of Health (2008) *A Portrait of Health. Key Results of the 2006/07 New Zealand Health Survey*. Wellington: Ministry of Health

[81] Ministry of Health (2008) *A Portrait of Health. Key Results of the 2006/07 New Zealand Health Survey*. Wellington: Ministry of Health

[82] Ministry of Health and Minister of Health (2008) *Health and Independence Report 2008*. Wellington: Ministry of Health

[83] Ministry of Health and Minister of Health (2008) *Health and Independence Report 2008*. Wellington: Ministry of Health

[84] Smith AH, Pearce NE. Determinants of differences in mortality between New Zealand Maoris and non- Maoris aged 15–64. N Z Med J. 1984; 97:101–108

[85] Westbrook I, Baxter J, Hogan J. Are Maori under-served for cardiac interventions? *N Z Med J*. 2001;114: 484–487.

[86] Harris, R et al (2006) *Effects of self-reported racial discrimination and deprivation on Maori health and inequalities in New Zealand: cross-sectional study*, The Lancet, Volume 367 Issue 9527

[87] http://www.nzdoctor.co.nz/news?article=1688BE03-EC23-4C78-889E-89297DFC515B

[88] Ministry of Health (2008) *A Portrait of Health. Key Results of the 2006/07 New Zealand Health Survey.* Wellington: Ministry of Health

[89] Ellison-Loschmann, L & Pearce, N (2006) *Improving Access to Health Care Among New Zealand's Maori Population* Am J Public Health. 2006 April; 96(4): 612–617

[90] Medical Council of New Zealand (2009) *The New Zealand Medical Workforce in 2008*

Chapter 4

[91] Pharmac (2007) *Prescription for Pharmacoeconomic Analysis – Methods for Cost Utility Analysis*, Pharmac

[92] http://www.nzma.org.nz/journal/119-1235/2014/

[93] Harper, P et al, (2003) *The challenge arising from the cost of haemophilia care: an audit of haemophilia treatment at Auckland Hospital*, Journal of the New Zealand Medical Association, 22-August-2003, Vol 116 No 1180

[94] NICE (2008) *Identifying and Supporting People Most at Risk of Dying Prematurely*

[95] Andriole, GL et al (2009) *Mortality Results from A Randomised Prostate Cancer Screening Trial* NEJM, 360;13

[96] Tengs et al (1995) *Five Hundred Life Saving Interventions and Their Cost Effectiveness*, Risk Analysis Vol 15 No3

[97] Martin, S et al (2008) *The link between health care spending and health outcomes for the new English Primary Care Trusts* University of York, CHE Research Paper 42

[98] Tengs et al (1995) *Five Hundred Life Saving Interventions and Their Cost Effectiveness*, Risk Analysis Vol 15 No3

[99] http://www.aafp.org/fpr/20041100/23.html

[100] Kizer, K.W. & Dudley, R.A. (2009) *Extreme Makeover: Transformation of the Veterans Health Care System* Annual Review of Public Health, Vol. 30, April 2009

[101] Starfield, Shi and Macinko, *Contribution of Primary Care to Health Systems and Health, The Milbank Quarterly*, Vol. 83, No. 3, 2005 (pp. 457–502)

[102] World Health Organisation (2000) *The World Health Report 2000: Health Systems: Improving Performance* Switzerland WHO

[103] Starfield, B (1998) *Primary care: balancing health needs, services and technology* New York: Oxford University Press

[104] http://www.newyorker.com/reporting/2009/06/01/090601fa_fact_gawande

[105] Cumming, J, Gribben, B (2007) *Evaluation of the Primary Health Care Strategy: Practice Data Analysis 2001-2005*, Victoria University of Wellington

[106] Ministry of Health (2008) *A Portrait of Health. Key Results of the 2006/07 New Zealand Health Survey*. Wellington: Ministry of Health

[107] Waldegrave, C (2009) *Healthy Families, Young Minds and Developing Brains: Enabling all Children to Reach Their Potential* Families Commission

[108] Merry et al *The CMDHB Infant Mental Health Project* CMDHB

[109] Lattice Consulting (undated) *The Evaluation of Community Living Services* CMDHB

[110] Russell, L (2009) *Preventing Chronic Disease: An Important Investment, But Don't Count on Cost Savings Health Affairs*, Volume 28, Number 1

[111] Goetzel, R (2009) *Do Prevention or Treatment Services Save Money? The Wrong Debate* Health Affairs Volume 28, No1

[112] Weel, C. van & Michels, J (1997) *Dying, not old age, to blame for costs of health care* Lancet v.350 p1159

[113] Bryant, J et al (2004) *Population Ageing and Government Health Expenditures in New Zealand*, 1951-2051 New Zealand Treasury Working Paper 04/14

[114] Le Fanu op. cit.

[115] Streat, S and Callaghan, *Limiting and Withdrawing Treatment*

[116] Le Fanu op. cit.

[117] Higginson I, Sen-Gupta GJA, *Place of Care in Advanced Cancer.* Journal of Palliative Medicine 2004;3 287-300

[118] Steinhauser, KE et al. *Factors considered important at the end-of-life by patients, family, physicians and other care providers* JAMA 2000;284 (19):2476-2482

[119] Heyland DK et al, *What matters most in end-of-life care: perceptions of seriously ill patients and their family members* CMAJ 2006; 174: 627-633

[120] Streat, S (2005) *When do we Stop?* Critical Care and Resuscitation 2005; 7: 227-232

[121] Murray, S et al (2005) *Illness Trajectories and Palliative Care* BMJ Volume 330 1007-1011.

Chapter 5

[122] From the Hippocratic Oath http://www.pbs.org/wgbh/nova/doctors/oath_modern.html

[123] Davis, K et al (2007) *Mirror, Mirror on the Wall: an International Update on the Comparative Performance of American Health Care* Commonwealth Fund

[124] http://www.fishnz.co.nz/481105la11.html

[125] Ministry of Health and Minister of Health (2008) *Health and Independence Report 2008.* Wellington: Ministry of Health

[126] Blakely, T, Pearce, N, (2002) *Socio-economic position is more than just NZDep,* NZ Med J 2002; 115: 109-11

[127] Ministry of Health (2008) *A Portrait of Health. Key Results of the 2006/07 New Zealand Health Survey.* Wellington: Ministry of Health

[128] Seddon, ME et al, (1999) *Waiting times and prioritisation for coronary artery bypass surgery in New Zealand* Heart; 81:586-592

[129] Hurst & Siciliani (2003) *Tackling Excessive Waiting Times for Elective Surgery: A Comparison of Policies in Twelve OECD countries,* OECD Health Working Paper 6

[130] CMDHB (2007) *Improving Access to Elective Surgery 1996/97 – 2005/06*

[131] Manning & Paterson (2005) *"Prioritization": Rationing Health Care in New Zealand,* Legislating and Litigating Health Care Rights Around the World, Winter 2005.

[132] Derived from Figure 6.2 in Roake J, "Managing Waiting Lists". In Gauld R, ed. *Continuity amid chaos: health care management and delivery in New Zealand.* Dunedin: University of Otago Press; 2003:107-121.

[133] Cardiac Surgery Service Development Working Group (2008) *Cardiac Surgery Services in New Zealand*

[134] http://www.cmdhb.org.nz/Funded-Services/General-Practice/Waiting-Times/default.htm#GeneralMedicine

[135] Cardiac Surgery Service Development Working Group (2008) *Cardiac Surgery Services in New Zealand*

[136] Pearce, J et al (2008) *Have Geographic Inequalities in Cause Specific Mortality in New Zealand Increased During the Period 1980-2001,* NZMJ 5 Sept 2008, Vol 121, No 1281

Chapter 6

[137] Treasury (2006) *New Zealand's Long-Term Fiscal Position*

[138] Treasury (2006) *New Zealand's Long-Term Fiscal Position*

[139] Parkin et al (1987) *Aggregate health care expenditures and national income. Is health care a luxury good?* J Health Econ. 1987 Jun;6(2):109-27

[140] Ministry of Health (2008), *Briefing for the Incoming Minister of Health*

[141] Treasury (2006) *New Zealand's Long-Term Fiscal Position*

[142] Bryant, J et al (2004) *Population Ageing and Government Health Expenditures in New Zealand, 1951-2051* New Zealand Treasury Working Paper 04/14

[143] Source ONS http://www.telegraph.co.uk/news/uknews/1576933/Britons-spend-one-fifth-of-income-on-homes.html

[144] Boden, W, Taggart, DP (2009) Diabetes with Coronary Disease – A Moving Target amid Evolving Therapies? NEJM 360; 24 June 11, 2009

[145] Raymont, A., Hospital discharges in New Zealand 1991-2005: changes over time and variation between districts. New Zealand Medical Journal, 2008. 121(1279)

[146] Congressional Budget Office (2008) *Technological Change and the Growth of Health Care Spending*

[147] http://www.ssc.govt.nz/display/document.asp?docid=6964&pageno=5#P391_17902

[148] Davis, K et al (2007) *Mirror, Mirror on the Wall: an International Update on the Comparative Performance of American Health Care* Commonwealth Fund

[149] Ministry of Health (2008), *Briefing for the Incoming Minister of Health*

[150] National Health Committee (2007) *Meeting the Needs of People with Chronic Conditions* Wellington

[151] World Economic Forum, Global Risks 2009

[152] National Health Committee (2007) *Meeting the Needs of People with Chronic Conditions* Wellington

[153] Ministry of Health (2008), *Briefing for the Incoming Minister of Health*

[154] Ministry of Health (2008), *Briefing for the Incoming Minister of Health*

[155] Goss, J (2008) *Projection of Australian health care expenditure by disease 2003 to 2033*, Australian Institute of Health and Welfare, Canberra

[156] PWC, (2007) *Diabetes New Zealand*

[157] Wanless, D (2004) *Securing Good Health for the Whole Population*, UK Treasury

[158] Davis, K et al (2007) *Mirror, Mirror on the Wall: an International Update on the Comparative Performance of American Health Care* Commonwealth Fund

Chapter 7

[159] Medical Reference Group, Health Workforce Advisory Committee. (2006) *Fit for Purpose and for Practice: Advice to the Minister of Health on the issues concerning the medical workforce in New Zealand.* Wellington: Health Workforce Advisory Committee.

[160] Medical Training Board (2009) *Annual Report*

[161] http://www.guide2.co.nz/politics/party-policies/national-party-doctor-training/9/3175

[162] Zurn, P & Dumont, JC (2008) *Health Workforce and International Migration: Can New Zealand Compete?* OECD Health Working Papers 33

[163] Workforce Taskforce (2007) *Reshaping Medical Education and Training to Meet the Challenges of the 21st Century*

[164] www.ers.dol.govt.nz/union/pdfs/Union-Membership-2006.pdf

[165] http://www.asms.org.nz/Site/News/Media_Statements_07/10_April_07.aspx

[166] http://tvnz.co.nz/content/53882

[167] http://www.nzherald.co.nz/health/news/article.cfm?c_id=204&objectid=10582478

[168] NZ Herald 3 Jan 2009

[169] Medical Council of New Zealand (2009) *The New Zealand Medical Workforce in 2008*

[170] SMO Commission (2009) *Senior Doctors in New Zealand: Securing the Future*

[171] Saturday July 14 2007 *Hospitals to Act on Soaring Locum Pay*

[172] Source Ministry of Health Outsourced Medical Costs

[173] Medical Council of New Zealand (2009) *The New Zealand Medical Workforce in 2008*

[174] OECD Health Data 2008, our calculations

[175] Yeoman, A & Parry, S (2007), *A survey of colonoscopy capacity in New Zealand's public hospitals* JNZMA Vol 120 No 1258

[176] Bodenheimer, T, Lorig, K, Holman, H et al, (2002) *Patient Self Management of Chronic Disease in Primary Care*, JAMA 2002;288(19): 2469-2475

[177] Donaldson, L (2003) *Expert Patients Usher in a New Era of Opportunity for the NHS* BMJ Volume 326 14 June

Chapter 8

[178] http://www.nzdoctor.co.nz/news?article=78f0a723-d35a-4683-be2b-4b58c08708c6

[179] Coster, GD (2004) *Health Needs Assessment: Impact on Planning and Purchasing in the Public Health Sector in New Zealand* Victoria University thesis

[180] D.C. Hadorn (1991), *Setting health care priorities in Oregon. Cost-effectiveness meets the Rule of Rescue,* JAMA 265, 2218-25.

[181] Medical Council of New Zealand (2009) *The New Zealand Medical Workforce in 2008*

[182] The Press 07/06/2007, page 2 and Ministry of Health locum cost figures, adjusted for population.

[183] Beasley R & Holt, S (2002) *The Burden of Asthma in New Zealand,* Asthma Foundation

[184] Jackson R & Broad, J (2003) *The Burden of COPD in New Zealand,* Asthma Foundation

[185] Garrett, J et al (2009) *A survey of respiratory services in New Zealand undertaken by the Thoracic Society of Australia and New Zealand (TSANZ)* NZMJ 13 February 2009, Vol 122 No 1289

[186] University of York (2008) The Link Between Health Care Spending and Health Outcomes for the New English Primary Care Trusts

[187] Raymont, A., Hospital discharges in New Zealand 1991-2005: changes over time and variation between districts. New Zealand Medical Journal, 2008. 121(1279)

[188] McCarthy, D et al (2009) Geisinger Health System: Achieving the Potential of System Integration Through Innovation, Leadership, Measurement, and Incentives; Commonwealth Fund pub. 1233 vol. 9

[189] Cumming, J, Gribben, B (2007) *Evaluation of the Primary Health Care Strategy: Practice Data Analysis 2001-2005,* Victoria University of Wellington

[190] http://www.numberwatch.co.uk/risks_of_travel.htm

[191] http://www.qic.health.govt.nz/moh.nsf/indexcm/qic-sentinel-and-serious-events-report-0708

[192] The Press 6 July 2006

[193] Soleimani, (2006) *Learning from mistakes in New Zealand hospitals: what else do we need besides "no-fault"?* NZMA Vol 119, No 1239

[194] Levitt & Dubner (2005) *Freakonomics: A Rogue Economist Explores the Hidden Side of Everything*, Harper Collins

[195] Le Fanu, J (1999) *The Rise and Fall of Modern Medicine*, Carroll & Graf, New York

[196] Ministerial Review Group (2009) *Meeting the Challenge*, Ministry of Health

[197] www.ihi.org

[198] Davis, K et al (2007) *Mirror, Mirror on the Wall: an International Update on the Comparative Performance of American Health Care* Commonwealth Fund

[199] Mays, N, Blick, G (2009) *How Can Primary Health Care Contribute Better to Health System Sustainabilty? A Treasury Perspective*, Health Section, State Sector Performance Group

[200] Cumming, J, Gribben, B (2007) *Evaluation of the Primary Health Care Strategy: Practice Data Analysis 2001-2005*, Victoria University of Wellington

Chapter 9

[201] Bohmer et al (2001) *Maxmising Health Gain Within Available Resources in the New Zealand public health system*; Health Policy 55

[202] Paul, C et al *Making policy decisions about population screening for breast cancer: The role of citizens' deliberation.* Health Policy, Volume 85, Issue 3, Pages 314-320

[203] Porter, M.E. & Teisberg, E.O. (2006) *Redefining Health Care: Creating Value-Based Competition on Results* Harvard Business Press

[204] Charles Kenney (2008) *The Best Practice: How the New Quality Movement is Transforming Medicine* PublicAffairs

[205] Gawande, A (2004) *The Bell Curve*, excerpt from the New Yorker December 6 2004.

[206] Mays, N (2006) *Use of Targets to Improve Health System Performance: NHS Experience and Implications for New Zealand* Treasury WP 06/06

[207] Ministry of Health and Minister of Health (2008) *Health and Independence Report 2008.* Wellington: Ministry of Health

[208] Source CMDHB, NZ Treasury presentation 22 May 2008

[209] Medical Training Board (2009), *The Future of the Medical Workforce*

[210] Reliability targets for Eagle Air

[211] http://www.radionz.co.nz/news/stories/2009/04/03/1245a957dc60

[212] Feachem, RGA, Sekhri, NK and White, KL (2002) Getting more for their dollar: a comparison of the NHS with California's Kaiser Permanente BMJ 2002;324:135-143 (19 January)

The following books by Gareth Morgan can be obtained from
http://shop.worldbybike.com/

**After the Panic, Surviving bad
investments and bad advice**
Gareth Morgan
2009 The Public Interest Publishing Company Ltd.

**Poles Apart - beyond the Shouting,
who's right about climate change?**
Gareth Morgan and John McCrystal
2009 Random House

Under African Skies
Jo and Gareth Morgan
2008 Random House

**KiwiSafer, how to keep your
money safe in KiwiSaver**
Gareth Morgan
2007 Random House

Backblocks America
Jo and Gareth Morgan
2007 Random House

Pension Panic
Gareth Morgan,
2006 Random House

Silkriders
Jo and Gareth Morgan
2006 Random House